# Praise for *Back in Control*

"*Back in Control*, by eminent spine surgeon David Hanscom, MD, is the perfect prescription for those suffering from chronic back pain. Dr. Hanscom's readable synthesis of frontier science and professional experience illuminates the functional interconnectivity of the spine, the nervous system, and the mind. This study reveals how perceived stress unconsciously sabotages our vitality; and, by following the described step-by-step processes, an "informed" consciousness can lead to mastery over one's health. *Back in Control* places one of the most powerful tools for self-healing into your very own hands. Read this powerful and wise prescription and reclaim sovereignty over your health and your life."
— **Bruce H. Lipton, PhD**, stem cell biologist and bestselling author of *The Biology of Belief, Spontaneous Evolution,* and *The Honeymoon Effect*

"*Back in Control* represents an innovative approach to chronic back pain, delivered by an extraordinary spine surgeon. No one should contemplate back surgery without first reading this book, as a cure may be closer than you think."
— **Howard Schubiner, MD,** author of *Unlearn Your Pain;* founder and director of the Mind-Body Medicine Center at St. John Providence Hospital, Southfield, MI

"Dr. Hanscom is a top Seattle spine surgeon who truly understands the how and why of back pain and sciatica. If your back's been hurting, this is the next book you should read."
— **David Tauben, MD,** Medical Director, Center for Pain Relief at University of Washington Medical Center-Roosevelt

"Dr. Hanscom's book contains a wealth of valuable insights for the majority of patients with chronic pain. Not only is the book insightful but it is also respectful of the suffering that patients with back pain experience. I am eager to recommend it to my back pain patients."
— **Jim Robinson, MD,** clinical professor, Center for Pain Relief at University of Washington Medical Center-Roosevelt

"As a society, we want (and need) the specialists who limit their practice to a specific body part of a system to treat people as whole people anyway—and to be alert to and provide basic services for problems in other parts or systems. It is *irresponsible* for any physician (or other health care practitioner) to ignore symptoms in any domain. An orthopedist like Dr. Hanscom who is alert to the possibility of psychosocial issues and attends to them is many people's dream of a wonderful doctor."
— **Jennifer Christian, MD,** Occupational Medicine; President of Webility; Founder of the Work Fitness and Disability Roundtable

"I have been treating patients with chronic pain for over 25 years. Since I have been working with David I have never seen patients experience such a decrease in their pain and improvement in their overall quality of life."
— **Suzanne Lacross, PhD,** clinical psychologist, Seattle, WA

"Dr. Hanscom addresses both the prevalent problem of unnecessary spine surgery and the lack of clarity regarding nonoperative care. I have the good fortune to work closely with him. His ideas have changed my approach to chronic pain. Our teamwork has given our patients tremendous reassurance knowing that their surgeon and their pain doctor are 'on the same page.'"
— **Joel Konikow, MD,** Swedish Hospital Pain and Headache Center, Seattle, WA

"In addition to being a great surgeon Dr. Hanscom is a great 'physiatrist.' I appreciate that he looks at a person as a whole and addresses issues of sleep, exercise, and the emotional aspects of pain as opposed to immediately relying on interventional procedures and surgeries."
— **Carolyn Marquardt, MD,** physiatrist, Bellevue, WA

"*Back in Control* has brought me new hope in dealing with a problem I believed I would suffer the rest of my life. Dr. Hanscom shares stories of his own personal saga of dealing with chronic pain. When he described the cycle of pain, anxiety, anger, victimhood, insomnia, and hopelessness, I felt relief for the first time in seven years—relief that I had finally found

someone who not only understood this interaction; but more importantly, had concrete tools and advice—proven techniques—for how to deal with it. I am recommending this book to all of my pain patients, and even those suffering emotional pain such as anxiety and depression. This man has walked in my shoes and I cannot thank him enough for writing such a readable, helpful, brilliant, cutting-edge book. You have given me hope!"
— **Diana Brady,** licensed marriage and family therapist, Sarasota, FL

"Dr. Hanscom's message is genuinely clear and heartfelt and he is an excellent communicator. He did a great job talking about his own journey into 'the Abyss' of the pain he suffered. This book has been a lifesaver. I have been in 'the Abyss' for over 7 years. Not any more with this great book. I see a light at the end of the tunnel."
— **Jim Green,** program director, WHPC Radio, Nassau Community College, Long Island, NY

"One word: life-changing! When I met Dr. Hanscom, I was a suffering skeptic: desperate and doubtful that anything could help my chronic pain. I found myself at the end of the line with doctors and treatments, all unable to provide a 'cure.' Yet, within 24 hours of meeting Dr. Hanscom, I began to feel the chains of chronic pain unshackle themselves, and for the first time in years, I felt hope. There are no magic pills or silver bullets. Dr. Hanscom will lead you on an introspective journey that takes work and commitment, but it's essential for anyone looking to take back their life. It's more than a title, it's an anthem. By reading this book and following Dr. Hanscom's suggestions, you too can be back in control."
— **Esty Gorman,** participant at Omega Institute, Rhinebeck, NY

"*Back in Control* has provided a key piece of my 4-way approach toward a pain-free life—without drugs, surgery or injections. Dr. Hanscom's colleagues at the University of Wisconsin Spine Clinic have high regard for his work and I feel more confident following his approach knowing that they agree that the mind-body link is essential to controlling chronic pain."
— **Steve Hauck**, engineer, Madison, WI

# David
# Hanscom
# MD

# BACK
# IN
# CONTROL

*A surgeon's roadmap
out of chronic pain*

Back In Control, 2nd Edition

Copyright © 2017 by David Hanscom, MD

Published by
Vertus Press
2515 4th Avenue #1701
Seattle, WA 98121

ISBN: 978-0-9882729-9-6
eISBN:978-0-9882729-8-9

Printed in the United States of America

Interior Design by GKS Creative

Cover Design by Alfio Cini

While all of the patient stories described in this book are based on true experiences, all of the names are pseudonyms, and some situations have been changed slightly for educational purposes and to protect each individual's privacy.

The information in this book is not offered, nor should it be used to treat or diagnose any particular disease or any particular patient. Neither the author nor the publisher is engaged in rendering professional advice or services to the individual reader.

Publisher's Cataloging-In-Publication Data

Names: Hanscom, David.
Title: Back in control : a surgeon's roadmap out of chronic pain / David Hanscom, MD.
Other Titles: Bac in control
Description: 2nd edition. | Seattle, WA : Vertus Press, [2016] | Includes bibliographical references.
Identifiers: ISBN 978-0-9882729-9-6 | ISBN 978-0-9882729-8-9 (ebook)
Subjects: LCSH: Backache--Treatment. | Chronic pain--Treatment. | Chronic pain--Psychological aspects. | Mind and body. | Spine--Surgery.
Classification: LCC RD771.B217 H36 2016 (print) | LCC RD771.B217 (ebook) | DDC 617.564/06--dc23

To my loving wife, Babs,
who supported me through this long journey.
Without her this book would not have been possible.

*Disease in man is never exactly the same as disease in an experimental animal, for in man the disease at once affects and is affected by what we call the emotional life. Thus the physician who attempts to take care of the patient while he neglects this factor is as unscientific as the investigator who neglects to control all of the conditions that affect his or her experiment... One of the essential qualities of the clinician is interest in humanity, for the secret of care is in caring for the patient.*

—FRANCIS PEABODY, MD
"The Care of the Patient"
*Journal of the American Medical Association*
March, 1927

# Contents

# Foreword

Much of my practice in spine surgery consists of giving a second opinion regarding the necessity of a proposed spine surgery. This chapter is written by a patient whom I saw once for a proposed surgery suggested by two other surgeons. He figured out most of his successful healing process on his own, and he wished to share his story.
—David Hanscom, MD

## My Journey Out of Pain
by Mark Owens

One early evening back in the summer of 2006, my neighbor Sam and I were riding horses out of the mountains near Libby, Montana. We'd been looking for grizzly bears high up in the Cabinet Mountain Wilderness and were done for the day. My horse Whiskey had been working hard for hours, and his cocked ears, snorts, and blows let me know that he wasn't happy about it. I urged him onward, anxious to get back to civilization before the night got too cold and dark.

Suddenly Whiskey dropped his head, stripped the reins from my left hand, and took off bucking down the boulder-strewn trail. On his fourth snap-roll, Whiskey launched me out of the saddle. "This is going to hurt," I remember thinking as I flew through the air. I had no idea how badly.

Just before I hit the ground, a log about eight inches in diameter caught me high up on my side, just under my left arm. My ribs—all of them on that side—cracked and then caved as they tried to rupture through the front wall of my chest. Almost immediately after my ribs gave way, my spine broke in two places. A tsunami of white-hot pain—the most intense I have ever known—shot through my body, as though I was being stabbed over and over again by a dozen daggers.

Sam went for help. By the time he got back to me and covered me with blankets, I'd been on the ground in the thirty-six-degree cold for five hours, wearing little more than jeans and a light shirt. Most of the heat in my body had escaped me; I was so numb that I couldn't even feel the warmth of the blankets.

An hour and a half after Sam arrived, seven men appeared, some on foot, others on horseback. They stuffed me in a heavy bivy sack and began carrying me, stumbling and falling on the dark, rocky trail. Our destination: a high alpine meadow one-and-a-half miles back up the mountain. At sunrise four-and-a-half hours later, we staggered into Moose Meadow, where all my bearers immediately fell asleep in the lush green grass. Finally, a Life Flight helicopter came and took me to the hospital in Kalispell, Montana.

There, surgeons fused a foot-long section of my spine by installing a ladder of titanium steel from my eighth thoracic to my second lumbar vertebrae. The next morning, two nurses stood me up to take my first post-surgical "walk," and I passed out from the pain. It was so extreme that nothing, not even a cocktail of morphine, OxyContin, oxycodone, and Norco were enough to quell it.

As I lay there going in and out of consciousness, I couldn't help but be in a state of disbelief. As a wildlife field biologist and conservationist, I'd worked in Africa with my wife Delia for 23 years in two of that continent's most remote wilderness areas. During my time there, I'd been charged by a number of animals: lions, elephants, Cape buffaloes, and some antelope. Poachers plotted to assassinate me in my camp and shot at my Cessna and helicopter. I'd also survived more than my share of near-misses while flying. Like most people speeding through life like a bullet on a mission, I felt almost invincible during all those years, and in 1996, I returned from Africa to the wilds of Idaho with hardly a scar. But that night high on a mountain above Libby, Montana, my luck had run out, and now I lay there bruised, broken, and vulnerable.

After a week, I was sent home from the hospital to begin my two-year-long recovery. With a crushed chest, a collapsed and re-inflated lung, and a veritable hardware store installed in my back, my pain levels ranged from six to ten for the first two months. Despite my efforts to limit the number of drugs I was taking, I was (unbeknownst to me) already becoming dependent on the suite of analgesics, sleep aids, muscle relaxants, and laxatives that had been prescribed for me. One night I took seven different drugs to help me sleep, not including vodka and Contac for colds. When I told this to my surgeon's nurse, she was surprised that I'd survived.

About six weeks post-surgery, my pain had dropped to about a level four. I was walking a mile a day and began trying to transition from prescription narcotics to over-the-counter drugs. But to my surprise I realized that I now had another problem to add to my recovery: I was addicted to my meds. Realizing this, I went "cold turkey" and was sleepless for ten days, cold sweats soaking my bed. Tremors made me jump and twitch all over for hours. I was finally able to sleep a little and manage my pain using over-the-counter drugs and a little vodka from time to time.

Two years after my surgery, I was considered fully recovered, yet I still felt as if I was carrying a chimpanzee on my back, its weight pressing me forward and making it impossible for me to stand up straight. My pain levels had crept back up to levels five to six most of the time, and my lower back was getting more painful, not less.

My body maintenance was nearly a full-time job: I hung from an inversion bed two to four times a day; I practiced yoga and did various other stretches; I lay across exercise balls, foam rollers, tennis balls, and a football. I walked two-to-four miles daily, did pull-ups in my doorway, lifted weights, danced, and did anything else I could do to keep moving. There was too little time for anything else and my career as a writer and field biologist was mostly moribund.

I was working hard to heal my body, but the truth was, I had descended into the perfect hell of acute chronic pain. In the years after my accident, I had stretches of times where I felt like I was healing, but for the most part, my pain was relentless: It attached itself to my body, mind, and spirit, sucking away my essence, a leech that was never sated and would never let go. It was a pain so severe that its spasms caused me to collapse onto dinner tables, to hold onto furniture so that I wouldn't fall as I moved about my home; a pain so all-consuming that it alienated some of my friends who couldn't stand to see me suffer. It was stupefying and isolating, crippling and confining. Over time, it literally caused my brain to shrink because I couldn't focus on anything else. It never forgave or forgot. It was the last to say goodnight and the first to greet me on waking in the morning. In the end, it made me want to die. I almost did, on purpose.

By 2012, six years after my accident, I again had so much pain in my lower back that I had another surgery to fuse L2 and L3. I had barely recovered from that when, driving with too little sleep and under the influence of muscle relaxers and sleep aids, I wrecked my truck and broke my back at L4.

By the spring of 2013, my legs were collapsing under me, I was holding onto furniture to keep from falling, and my pain levels were constantly between eight and ten. I began looking for another surgeon who could release me from this hell, and I found one in eastern Washington who explained that he had been a General Motors auto engineer before going to medical school.

"Your back has seen too much trauma," he said. "You really don't have any good options, and most of them would not relieve you of your pain or improve your range of motion. The only hope for you is what I call the Blue Plate Special." He went on to explain a two-day surgery during which he and another surgeon would filet me like a salmon, incising me from my clavicle to my pelvis in order to remove the titanium steel hardware that was buried in the straight, stiff fusion mass that spanned from the 8th thoracic to the 2nd lumbar vertebra. After breaking my spine through the fusion in two places, they would then replace the existing construct with a longer, more curved one that would better conform to the natural curvature of my original spine. Finally, they would remove calcium deposits (stenosis) in my spinal canal and extend the fusion to my pelvis. Most of my spine would become one solid piece of bone and hardware.

He presented all of this with what seemed to me to be fairly unrestrained glee, confidence bordering on over-confidence, and an air of certitude that defied his words when he said, "This will be quite a complicated surgery with a fair amount of risk and a long recovery, but frankly, any more conservative surgical options are bound to fail, leaving you worse off than you are now."

This wasn't the first time a surgeon had recommended this type of radical operation to me: before my fusion in 2012, another doctor had proposed something similar. Still, to hear it again was tough. At that point my mood could best be described as somber; his words were like lead weights pulling my head under water for the last time. He was so good at selling this surgery, however, that I felt strongly inclined to sign up for it right there and then, especially when he said that he could schedule the procedure within six weeks of that date. But in the end I left, telling him I'd have to think it over.

I walked out with the friend who was with me and before we even got to the parking lot, it hit me. I couldn't just go by this doctor's word for such a drastic procedure. I turned to my friend and said, "What if this is more about ego than what would be good for me? I need another opinion."

Two days later we entered the office of Dr. David Hanscom at the Swedish Medical Center in Seattle. Seconds after coming through the door he announced: "I've looked at the images of your back and I'm afraid

I cannot recommend you for surgery. I don't see a one-to-one correspondence between any dysfunction in your spine and the pain you are experiencing."

My mouth fell open in shock. Dr. Hanscom went on to explain that only about 20-30 percent of fusion surgeries for low back pain are successful, meaning that 70-80 percent are not. Furthermore, many of these surgeries leave patients worse off than they were before.

"Not only are they not successful," David explained, "but the fusion results in more force being placed on the healthy vertebrae above and below it, causing them to break down. Subsequent fusion surgeries may be needed every few years to lengthen the construct. Because of this, I quit performing spinal fusion surgeries for low back pain about twelve years ago. Nowadays, I do them only where I can identify a structural problem in the spine that is directly and obviously causing the pain. In your case I see nothing of the sort."

I felt strangely deflated and disoriented—as though I'd been given bad news, not good.

"But what am I supposed to do? I am not imagining this pain, that my legs are collapsing."

Dr. Hanscom agreed: "Your pain is real, it's just not coming from your spine."

"But my back is a mess; it must be causing my pain." Like so many other chronic back-pain sufferers, I could feel myself growing desperate to be sliced and diced because I had been programmed by ten different surgeons to believe that this was my only option.

"Actually, I've seen many backs much worse than yours. And in fact yours shows some wear and tear, but it is quite stable and nothing in your images suggests that it is causing your pain."

"You don't understand, Dr. Hanscom, I cannot live with this level of pain."

"Actually, I do understand," he replied. "Eighteen years ago I was much worse off than you. I was experiencing such severe chronic back pain and was so depressed that I was suicidal. My career, my marriage, my friendships—everything was in shambles. My life as I had known it was over."

I looked at this athletic and healthy man standing before me and could scarcely believe what he was telling me.

"But how..."

"I think you are suffering from what we call neurophysiologic disorder (NPD). Your brain is creating its own endogenous pain stimuli, rather like it does with phantom limb pain, registering pain even though the offending appendage has been removed." David went on to explain that research in neuroscience has confirmed that after about three months, chronic pain sufferers' brains are rewired with neural connections to newly developed brain centers that generate their own pain signals. These signals are independent of any dysfunction in the body below the victim's head.

I was candid with the doctor: I wasn't convinced. "To be honest, this sounds a little like snake oil to me," I said.

"Well, you can choose to go under the knife again with all of its associated risks and limitations, or you can read my book and learn about using simple techniques that even a grade-schooler can master, and maybe rid yourself of your chronic pain forever. You can start right away with 'expressive writing.' You simply spend fifteen to thirty minutes in the morning and again at night, writing down, in longhand, any thought that comes into your head. After you've written out each one in graphic and descriptive language, you immediately tear it up. Neurological research has shown that this creates a separation between the brain and the thought, so that you can begin re-training your brain to lay down new more positive neural pathways that wire around the old destructive ones. Some people experience remarkable pain relief almost right away, and some actually get rid of their pain altogether. Maybe you will be one of the lucky ones."

David then invited me to a "Rewire Your Brain" workshop being held at the Omega Center in Rhinebeck, New York, about three weeks later.

My friend and I left David's office feeling that this was too good to be true, but I was also resolved to try this "Neurophysiologic Disorder" approach to pain control before submitting to radical surgery. We drove south along the coast from Seattle, found a motel for the night, and I immediately tried my hand at expressive writing. I was quite sure it would never work for me.   David explained that different types of expressive writing, as well as other techniques used in his program, are being supported by a growing body of peer-reviewed scientific research, but I had not yet seen this work. As a scientist, I am skeptical by nature. Nonetheless, at that point I was willing to give anything a try.

The next morning when I awoke, I noticed that my lower back hadn't greeted me with a shot of pain before I even moved my legs to get up from bed, something that had occurred for years.

"No way; this cannot be," I said to myself as I stretched out my legs, fully expecting the usual lightning bolt of pain. But all I felt was a comparatively mild discomfort. I stood up and walked to the bathroom. Yes, it hurt as I walked, but nothing like it had since my accident in 2006. Still, I refused to credit the writing I had done.

We drove on into Oregon that day, and by late afternoon found ourselves lying on a nearly deserted beach with our heads on a chunk of driftwood, watching gulls wheeling overhead as the surf caressed our feet.

"I am afraid to believe this," I said to my friend, "but for the very first time in nine years I am virtually pain-free—and happy. It's as if a veil of agony has lifted from my face and I can see the world clearly again." I estimated that over the course of just less than two days I had somehow gotten rid of about 80 percent of my chronic pain.

It took me a while to trust this sudden release from the hell of chronic pain, but today, over a year later, I am going as much as an entire week at a stretch without needing to take any analgesics at all, not even Tylenol. Gradually my world has expanded again, and as I write this, I am planning a horseback ride back up the Cedar Creek trail where I nearly died nine years ago. It has become a regular pilgrimage for me, I think because I still cannot fully comprehend how I managed to escape the grip of soul-destroying chronic pain that so many others are enduring—many of them needlessly. If you are one of them, read on: this book will save your life. I know, because it surely saved mine.

We are on the cusp of a revolution in treating chronic pain, whether it is emotional or physical. Dr. David Hanscom and his colleagues in this pioneering effort are risking a great deal and sacrificing much to lead the charge against the profit-oriented medical establishment in promoting a treatment that costs nothing more than a little time, commitment, and the price of a notebook and a pencil. Oh yes, and the suspension of disbelief.

David and his cohorts are truly modern day heroes in this struggle.
—Mark Owens

# INTRODUCTION

## My Journey Out of Pain

I began my practice in orthopedic spine surgery in Seattle, Washington, in 1986. As I write this, it is my thirtieth year of being a complex-deformity spine surgeon. I completed my spine training in an internationally-acclaimed spine center in Minneapolis, Minnesota. It required an intensely focused, sustained effort to achieve that level of success. I was not only up to it, I wanted more. Then the wheels came off, and quickly.

My journey into chronic pain began after I had been in practice for a couple of years and it lasted over fifteen years. Initially, I had no idea what was happening. Until then, I had no hint of a problem—at least not one that I recognized. I didn't become a major complex spine surgeon by having anxiety. I was bulletproof. But then I began to sweat during surgery, something that had never occurred before, and by 1990, I was experiencing panic attacks. I pursued every possible avenue of treatment with a full medical and surgical workup. I went to psychotherapy, took medications, read every self-help book I could get my hands on, and attended workshops; yet I continued to spiral downward. By 1997, I had developed sixteen symptoms of what you will learn to recognize as NPD (neurophysiologic disorder), including a severe case of obsessive-compulsive disorder (OCD).

In 2002, I happened to pick up a book that recommended doing some simple expressive writing exercises, which involved getting any thoughts onto paper and tearing them up. I did the exercises, and within two weeks I began to pull out of my tailspin. Six months later, all of my sixteen symptoms had essentially disappeared, as I learned and practiced more of the concepts you will read about.[1]

I have been given a "gift" of extreme suffering that I would choose not to accept again. But I can look any patient in the eye and say, "Look, you may be suffering as much as I did, but not more. I do know what you are going through and it is a huge problem."

It took me another five years to sort out what had happened to me and be able to share what I'd learned with my patients. It wasn't until 2011 that I found out that what I'd been suffering from was an over-adrenalized nervous system with each organ in my body responding in its own way.[2]

I have now watched hundreds of patients become pain free much more quickly than I did. The most rewarding part of my practice has become to help people without hope successfully resolve their pain. A few people require surgery but most do not.

## The Chronic Pain Patient's Dilemma

The essence of the chronic pain problem is often that no one can find the source of your pain and no one believes you. Your suffering is severe and often extreme and there does not seem to be a way out. It's an extremely dark place to live in; for most, it's beyond comprehension.

Chronic pain cuts a wide swath. My patients often suffer a great deal, not only from chronic pain but also from the related anxiety and frustration. Their smiles are gone. Their family lives tend to be strained. Family members, instead of serving as a major source of support, are just trying to survive the emotional fallout from their loved one's distress. You might be labeled by friends, family, employers, claims examiners, and physicians as being unmotivated, seeking medications, malingering, and so on. Once you've been labeled, people can no longer see who you are, much less hear you and try to meet your needs. It's common, if not the rule, for sufferers to become socially isolated.

This isolation is just one of many stress factors that those in chronic pain must contend with. It's no news that stress affects our health and overall well-being in a major way, but the current medical system has not been set up to help patients deal with stress and it does not reward doctors for the time they spend talking to patients and coordinating their care.

In the chronic pain experience, the nervous system is firing on all cylinders, drastically magnifying pain impulses. These impulses course through the brain and nervous system over and over on a continuous loop. The more pain you experience, the more the impulses are magnified, and vice versa. Eventually these "circuits" are memorized, leading to a vicious circle that can be set off by even the slightest stimulus.

## Why Aren't the Solutions More Available?

Mainstream medicine doesn't have the correct diagnosis for chronic pain; that's why medical training doesn't teach physicians effective treatments. Instead, the profession is focused on finding a structural reason for every symptom, while it's 99 percent more likely that your physical symptoms are arising from physiological responses to the environment. This concept has actually been known for many centuries, dating back to Hippocrates. But the technology explosion combined with the business of medicine has railroaded this approach.

I wasn't taught anything about chronic pain or comprehensive rehab in medical school, nor at any point during my residencies or fellowships. I was taught that back pain disappears 90 percent of the time and that patients should just buy time until it resolves. I recall a conversation I had with a veteran orthopedic surgeon during my first year of practice. "You do a little of this and a little of that, and eventually the pain goes away," he said. What I didn't realize for many years was that it was the patients who went away when they became tired of not getting better with such random treatments.

It's unclear why I wasn't instructed in systematically treating the known variables that affect pain since they have been documented in thousands of research papers over the last fifty years. The literature shows that stressors like marital problems, difficulty at work, financial issues, amd more, are better predictors of how well a patient will recover from back surgery than the actual pathology that is being operated on.

The medical system is beginning to come around to these concepts but probably not at a rate that will help you. My main goal in this book is to give you enough information so that you can develop your own resources. It's necessary to be proactive with your health care providers. Not only are physicians not trained in the concept of continuity of care, insurance plans will usually not adequately pay for the resources needed to help you resolve your chronic pain. In fact, the medical world is so procedurally oriented that you will usually get moved from treatment to treatment without any continuity at all. Your anxiety and frustration will intensify, which will increase your pain. If you are in this state of mind you are not in a good place to make a decision about major spine surgery.

## The DOC Program

In this book I approach the chronic pain experience differently than most people in the health care industry, especially in its surgical arm. The difference is this: You must address all the variables that affect your perception of pain, especially those associated with calming down the nervous system, in order to heal. *Back in Control* reveals the way to calm a turbo-charged central nervous system.

Typically, when patients come to see me they've been bounced around the medical industry and their care is completely disorganized. They've usually had some combination of medication and physical therapy, but there's been no follow-up by the health care system. They're sleep-deprived, anxious, and barely able to function. They're also angry that the medical profession hasn't found a source of their pain and that there's no solution to their severe health problem.

As this book progresses, you will see that the essence of the problem is that Western medicine has medicalized a neurological disorder. Through my own experience of escaping chronic pain, learning from my patients and colleagues, and reading the medical literature on pain, a largely self-directed approach has emerged that I call the "DOC" (Define your Own Care) program.

The DOC program evolved when I was living in Sun Valley, Idaho. I'd gone from performing complex spine surgery at a major medical center to being a primary care spine doctor in a small town. I was well aware of the risk factors for developing chronic pain and could tell within a few minutes who needed a more intense approach.

I discovered that by providing a systematic approach to dealing with all aspects of a pain problem, I could almost always help patients become more functional. But more surprising to me was that, not only would they become more functional, many would experience a nearly complete recovery. Patients who had been disabled for quite a while would have a remarkable improvement in their pain, off narcotics, and resume an almost normal lifestyle. Frequently the new lifestyle was more active and satisfying than anything they had experienced before. I had not anticipated that type of response.

The DOC program shifts the focus from searching for the pain source, which may not even be identifiable on a test, to what you can do to become more functional. It addresses all the factors contributing to chronic pain and a turbocharged nervous system—lack of sleep, anxiety, medications, goal setting, physical conditioning, and anger—and goes through the best way to deal with them, one by one. For the outcome to be successful, each component must be carefully treated.

Since the medical establishment is not set up to take a comprehensive approach to your care, it's crucial to take your care into your own hands. This program shows you how to fill in the gaps left by automatically or randomly assigned treatments and also tells you when to insist on adequate follow-up by your health care providers. It's a much better approach than simply waiting to be told what to do.

## Esty

In 2013, Dr. Fred Luskin, a Stanford psychologist, my wife, Babs Yohai, and I held a five-day workshop at the Omega Institute in Rhinebeck, New York. One of the participants was a thirty-two-year-old woman named Esty, who had been experiencing severe neck pain for four years. She'd seen ten physicians, undergone six neck injections, and was on daily narcotics. She was still working in marketing but struggling to stay on her feet. She was not in a good mood. We set up the seminar around structure, hope, forgiveness, and play. You'll see how these are relevant as you progress through this book. She was in so much pain that I did not have any expectations that our workshop would help her. She sat through the first day grabbing her neck the entire day but, that night she began doing expressive writing.

Dr. Luskin, who is also the author of *Forgive for Good*,[3] was brilliant at explaining forgiveness. My wife, Babs, a professional tap dancer, took us through some simple rhythms and we all just began to laugh. I personally have no capacity to deal with rhythm. By the end of the week, Esty was free of pain, and she is still active and thriving without pain—and without medications. Here is her last email, about three years after the Omega week.

> *Dear David, Of course I'm okay with my story being told. Things have been a bit crazy over the past two weeks, not only did I purchase my first house, celebrate a birthday, but I also JUST GOT ENGAGED!!! Talk about bringing that mood board to life!! :) I wouldn't be doing any of this if it weren't for your team, or at*

*the very least, I wouldn't be able to enjoy every moment as much as I am, and I am so thankful to you coming into my life and making such an incredible impact. Give Babs a huge hug for me, talk soon! Esty :)*

Many other Omega participants have experienced similar levels of healing. I see people weekly in my clinic who are not only pain-free, but they are also thriving at a level they never imagined possible. Not only does the pain decrease but also their anxiety drops. I come out of my clinic every day inspired by my patients' will and determination. All of us want to remain in control of our destiny and live a life full of joy and creativity. It is incredibly rewarding watching my patients reconnect with that energy.

## Putting DOC into Action

Reading this book is not going to resolve your pain. It's only a framework to help you understand the neurological nature of chronic pain and various factors that affect your perception of it. You will then be able to find your own solution. It is not difficult, but you have to actively engage with the process to experience freedom from your pain.

The DOC process includes some of the following strategies you can use to solve chronic pain:

- Separate from anxiety by breaking the cycle of negative thoughts.
- Identify stress-inducing anger triggers.
- Give up victim status.
- Become more proactive about your care.
- Understand your medications so you can make better decisions with your doctor about how to optimize them and minimize their side effects.
- Create a vision for recovery and living a productive life.

The program is intended to be implemented in partnership with anyone involved in your care, including your physician, pain psychologist, physiatrist, physical therapist, or chiropractor. Think of it as a team set up to work on each part of your recovery.

You may be thinking, "I've tried medication! I've done stress management! I still have pain!" It's true that you may have already tried one or more of the parts of this program. But it's the step-by-step, structured combination of addressing *all* the aspects of pain, with *you* in charge, that will make an impact on your quality of life.

## Not Doing Surgery

All this is now coming full circle. In my first book, I stated that if a patient had a surgical issue and was experiencing chronic pain, it should be dealt with immediately. My reasoning was that the nervous system was fired up and that the patient could not tolerate much more pain. So, when presented with a scenario like that, I was more aggressive performing surgery. It turns out that my thinking was flawed. Performing surgery in the presence of an over-adrenalized nervous system yielded inconsistent results, and patients often had more pain after a technically well-executed operation. I was perplexed.

A few years ago, my team pointed out that when the surgical patients engaged in a structured rehab program, such as using the DOC process, post-operative pain was reduced, rehab was easier, and outcomes were consistently better. I implemented a protocol for all our patients undergoing elective surgery. Patients had to be:

- Aware of the nature of chronic pain
- Sleeping reasonably well
- On a stable medication program
- Feeling some abatement of their anxiety and anger
- Working to become more physically active.

We require at least 8–12 weeks of full engagement in this protocol before performing elective surgery. What happened has been completely unexpected. I am seeing patient after patient come in for their final pre-operative visit and cancel surgery because their pain has either significantly improved or disappeared. As their mood and sleep improved the pain abated. It has become problematic in that I have lost a significant part of my surgical practice. I have now witnessed over fifty patients with severe structural problems become pain free. At the same time, it has also been incredibly rewarding to watch my patients enter a new life without the risk of surgery. I can assure you that after thirty years of performing and observing spine surgery, the risks are real, and failed surgery can destroy a person's life.

In the first edition of this book, published in 2012, I focused almost entirely on back pain and spine surgery. But, because the principles I present in this new book apply to all parts of the body, I have expanded my focus to include any kind of chronic pain. And, now that we know how big a role our emotions play in the creation and persistence of physical pain, we must include all these factors in a successful treatment approach.

I am happy to share with you the successful strategies I discovered during my fifteen-year struggle with chronic pain. Welcome to your new life!

# SECTION 1:
# DESCENT INTO THE ABYSS

# CHAPTER 1

---

# The Pathway into Chronic Pain

IF YOU ARE EXPERIENCING ANY TYPE OF CHRONIC PAIN, it's probably safe to say that this is not how you expected your life to turn out. You likely didn't envision this state of affairs on the day you graduated from high school. You didn't foresee a future where you'd have unrelenting pain for months or even years. You didn't imagine that it would be hard to get out of bed day in and day out. You didn't think you'd be irritable with loved ones and friends, or they might start to avoid you. Your pain crept up on you without warning—and now you're in one of the worst situations that exists in the human experience. You're in a nightmare that affects every aspect of your life, seemingly without means of escape. What happened to your dreams?

I am an orthopedic spinal deformity surgeon who specializes in complex spinal problems in all areas of the spine, from the neck to the pelvis. Most of my patients are in chronic pain, and much of my practice is spent helping them become free of it, with or without surgery. I spend a great deal of time addressing a condition called "failed back syndrome." This term describes what happens to patients who have undergone multiple spinal surgeries that have failed. In many of these cases, the spine breaks down around a fusion that often did not need to be done, resulting in a major deformity. Patients are much worse off, and the revision surgeries have high rates of major complications. It is a huge tragedy that destroys people's lives.

I have personally experienced chronic pain, starting years ago during my first year of orthopedic surgery residency in Hawaii. One day when I was jogging, I felt a burning sensation on the soles of my feet, which continued during subsequent jogs. My ears began to ring as well, but I simply chose to ignore all of it. I attributed the burning to running on hot pavement and the ringing to having worked in heavy construction without ear protection. Little did I know that within five years, I would have a fully-developed chronic pain syndrome, with no idea what had hit me or how to fix it. I'd had no instruction regarding the nature of chronic pain at any point in my training. My ordeal lasted over twenty years, and the last seven were practically intolerable. Miraculously, I pulled out of it in 2003, but it took me another few years to understand what had happened to me and how I escaped this level of suffering. This book is based on my personal experience with chronic pain, my work with patients, and breakthrough discoveries from the research literature.

I have witnessed hundreds of patients who had been in total agony become pain-free with the correct diagnosis and treatment approach. The correct diagnosis is that chronic pain is a *maladaptive neuropathological disease state*, a condition that is created and exacerbated by a multitude of factors.[1,2,3] With this book you will come to recognize that condition and learn simple, non-intrusive remedies that are extremely effective in treating it.

The roadmap out of chronic pain consists of three steps:

1. Understanding that chronic pain is caused by both physical and emotional factors
2. Treating all contributing factors simultaneously
3. Taking charge of your own care

## The Neurophysiological Basis of Chronic Pain

We'll explore the connection between chronic pain and the nervous system. The descriptive term, "neurophysiological," is a combination of the words "neurological," the structure and function of the nervous system; and "physiology," defined as the ways that living things or any of their parts function.

How does the body depend on the nervous system? The body has to receive and interpret input from the environment through its various nervous system receptors before it physiologically responds in a way to ensure survival. Each signal is processed as pleasant, unpleasant, or neutral. All these signals are constantly competing with each other, creating an ever-changing chemical cocktail. The nervous system receptors connect with your brain to form your senses, which include:

- Taste
- Sound
- Smell
- Vision
- Touch
    - Light touch and pressure
    - Sharp or dull
    - Hot or cold
- Numerous other receptors supplying feedback about thirst, hunger, the position of your body in space, etc.

Some receptors are concentrated in one area, such as in your ears, nose, tongue, and eyes. Others are spread throughout your body, as are the touch and position receptors. But receptors have no inherent capacity to experience sensation—that is, they cannot "feel"; rather, receptors send signals through the peripheral nervous system to your brain, which interprets them. For example, when you touch something hot, the feeling of heat isn't in your finger; it's in your brain. A person who experienced a stroke in the brain's occipital lobe—the area responsible for vision—may be blinded, in spite of the fact that the person's eyes are still fully functional. Sensations are not experienced if they're not processed by your brain.

As the peripheral receptors send billions of impulses per second to the central nervous system (brain and spinal cord), they are interpreted every millisecond by what I call the "junction box"—the sum total of all the nervous system's activity at a given moment. Your body will interpret the net output of the junction box as pleasant, unpleasant, or neutral. How you react to this output matters enormously. Your body will chemically and emotionally respond with reward chemicals for net pleasant input and stress chemicals for negative input.

Reward chemicals include oxytocin (the love drug), dopamine, and Valium-type relaxing ones. They allow you to feel content, relaxed, happy, excited, etc. Stress chemicals include adrenaline and cortisol. They signal danger and cause you to feel anxious. Thus, your behavior is guided by your net chemical environment; you will gravitate toward reward hormones and avoid stress-related ones.

Depending on the intensity and duration of unpleasant sensory input, there is a progression of negative emotions that goes like this:

- Alert
- Nervous
- Anxious
- Afraid
- Paranoid
- Terrorized

When you feel emotions, what you are feeling is the effect of chemicals acting on your body's organs. Therefore, anxiety is the body's chemical reaction to stress. It's a feeling deeply rooted in survival that humans go to great lengths to avoid. A high level of sustained anxiety is intolerable.

In our bodies, a malfunction becomes disruptive only when it interferes with function enough to elicit a physiological response. For example, a person may have a superficial ulcer in their stomach that's not causing any problems. If it erodes through the stomach wall, however, it will cause inflammation and pain.

Conversely, you may have no anatomical problem, but you feel pain nonetheless—possibly because your body is reacting to a stressful situation. For instance, if you are yelled at by your boss or coworker, your body will respond with adrenaline and other stress chemicals. Adrenaline decreases the blood supply to your stomach, so you might have a stomachache. In other words, you will experience physical symptoms without any change in the structure of your digestive tract. The symptoms usually will resolve after the situation cools down—unless you keep thinking about it.

When you are exposed to any unpleasant sensation, you will take action to either eliminate the source of the pain or avoid it. If you are hungry, you will eat. If your hand is over a hot flame, you will pull it away. You don't go down dark alleyways. Your behavior, based on preventing an unfavorable chemical environment in your body, allows you to survive. [3]

### *Thoughts Are Sensory Input*

Thoughts elicit the same chemical responses as any other sensations. The responses can be pleasant, neutral, or unpleasant, with corresponding results very similar to other kinds of sensory input. Using functional MRIs (fMRIs), which reveal the effects of stimuli on different areas of the brain, researchers have discovered that physical and emotional pain activate similar regions of the brain. [4,5]

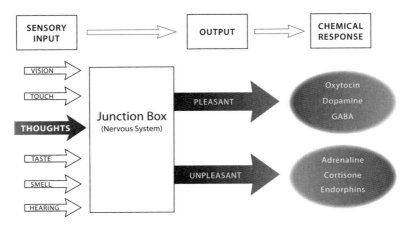

*Chemical Response to Sensory Input*

With these functional MRI scans, a labeled sugar, glucose (the brain's fuel), is injected intravenously and travels to metabolically active areas of the brain. Sophisticated imaging advances allow researchers to see increasingly specific areas of activity in response to various sensory inputs, as well as detailed patterns. So, thoughts are your mental link to the environment, similar to other sensations, which are physical links that allow you to protect yourself and thrive. Although the patterns of activity are different, the involved areas of the brain are similar. Emotional pain is equivalent to physical pain, especially when it comes to the body's chemical response. [6]

The major difference between thoughts and other sensory input is that you cannot escape from the former. All the other sensory input, such as taste, smell, and touch can be avoided or controlled. Neither of these strategies is effective in controlling unconstructive repetitive thoughts (URTs). The more you attempt to avoid or control them, the stronger they become.[7] The result is that your body becomes full of stress hormones and is under a sustained adrenaline/cortisol assault. The effects of adrenaline include a racing pulse, perspiring, decreased reasoning capacity, slowing of the digestive system, increased inflammatory response, compromised immune system, and dilated airways, in addition to experiencing anxiety. The collective effects of these inputs can become overwhelming. It's an enormous problem and at some point, people simply become ill. It can be compared to driving your car down the freeway in first or second gear with the engine racing. Your body and mind will eventually break down. The link between stress and disease has been well-documented. [8]

Combining my personal experience of suffering from chronic pain and treating thousands of patients with this last decade of neuroscience research, I firmly believe that the sustained release of stress hormones, brought on by the progressive intensity of URTs, is the primary cause and driver of chronic pain.

Chronic anxiety begins early in life for many people. My migraines began when I was five. Young children and teens are increasingly suffering from chronic mental and physical pain at younger ages. A 2015 paper reported that there were 1.7 million children in the U.S. alone suffering from chronic pain with an annual estimated cost of 19.5 billion dollars. [9]

Since you cannot escape unconstructive repetitive thoughts (URTs) and are not taught at a societal level how to process them, it seems that they are the logical driving force in the creation of chronic pain. Your organ systems respond to these in their own specific ways (described in detail in Chapter 2), creating any number of physical symptoms.[10]

If you have pre-existing anxiety and then are injured, there is a higher chance your resulting pain will become chronic because the pain circuits are already fired up.[11] It is well-documented that risk factors for developing chronic pain include anxiety, catastrophizing, insomnia, depression, and pre-existing chronic pain in any part of your body. Neuroscientists have a saying: "Neurons that fire together, wire together."

### *Emotional and Physical Pain Are Equivalent*

As stated above, research has revealed that there is a significant overlap between the neurological patterns of emotional and physical pain. A landmark fMRI study performed in 2003 showed that similar areas of the brain were activated during a simulated social rejection scenario (emotional pain) and the application of a heat wand to the volunteer's forearm (physical pain).[4]

The participants were asked to lie in an fMRI machine. They then participated in a computer game of three-way catch. The computer was programmed to suddenly exclude them from the game, and when that happened, researchers saw that neurological circuits lit up in the area of the brain that was activated when the heat wand was applied to the subject's arm. Humans have long used the phrase, "You hurt my feelings." This experiment validates that physical and mental pain share similar brain circuitry.

Now let's look at the pain-brain interaction more closely. Pain has at least two parts: The "somatosensory component" localizes the pain to the specific body part, while the affective component provides an emotional response. The two components activate two different areas of brain circuitry. When you experience physical pain, both the somatosensory and affective areas are active. It would make sense that you would not be that happy about being in pain. When you experience emotional pain, such as being rejected, research has shown that only the affective component lights up. (As was the case with the three-way catch exclusion game, above.) Why would your physical pain centers become active if only your feelings are hurt?

But wait. Researchers are now questioning whether the emotional pain created in the research setting was strong enough to detect this possibility. Instead of just being left out of playing a computerized game of catch, the experiment was repeated with the volunteers visualizing a time when a person had just broken off a close relationship with them. Guess what? The physical pain centers lit up in addition to the predicted emotional pain centers. The overlap between emotional and physical pain is greater than originally thought. The research is progressing rapidly and more details will surely be uncovered.

A review paper written by Dr. Eisenberger, a physician who conducted the original 2003 research at UCLA, lays out some more important findings. These findings come from several research centers using similar approaches with fMRIs and other increasingly sophisticated ways to measure brain activity:[5]

- Factors that increase social pain will increase physical pain. When you are upset for any reason, your brain will be more reactive in the areas reflecting physical distress. This is just brain activity and does not account for the increased sensitivity of your nervous system when bathed in stress chemicals. In animal studies, it has been shown that nerve conduction increases by 30–40 percent. That would make sense from a survival perspective in that you would want to have your senses as heightened as much as possible when there is a potential threat. [12]
- Factors that increase physical pain will increase social pain. We all know that when we don't physically feel well we are more reactive to those around us. Our feelings are hurt more easily and we may get upset. Indeed, researchers have documented this phenomenon in the lab by creating an inflammatory reaction by injecting an inciting agent. Unfortunately, I see part of this played out in my office when I talk to the family members of patients in pain. No one is happy on a bad day. When you are in pain and upset, there is high chance that you are not being nice to those close to you. They deserve better.
- Factors that decrease social pain will decrease physical pain.

Social support has long been known to help in healing and decreasing pain in many arenas. However, it has now been shown on fMRIs to directly decrease the activity of the pain circuits in the brain. This has been demonstrated by measuring activity when volunteers look at a picture of a stranger versus when they look at an image of a loved one.

• Factors that decrease physical pain will decrease social pain. As you can see, all these factors are interrelated. Again, as documented in the research setting, you will mentally feel better when you have less pain and are in a better mood. By consistently creating a supportive social network and becoming happier, your pain will decrease and you will feel better. Unfortunately, patients in pain tend to endlessly complain about their troubles to anyone who will listen. The people most apt to engage in this conversation are those who are also in pain. Talk about reinforcing negative pathways!

Dr. Eisenberger's summary of the problem is compelling. She points out that the consequences of social pain are potentially as damaging as physical pain. How absurd is it that it is not socially tolerated to physically assault someone but somehow verbal abuse and rejecting someone is more acceptable? [13] We already know how this kind of situation plays out, as many medical studies have documented the devastation caused by abuse of any kind. Even neglect is problematic in that it is a form of social rejection. [14]

## Anxiety, Power, and Bullying

To be connected to other people is one of the strongest human drives. Humans evolved by interacting with other humans. We also have a deep need for acceptance. This sets up a serious contradiction because our even deeper need is to avoid anxiety.

We try to avoid anxiety, or—if we already have it—we try to get rid of it. One common method we use is to increase our sense of control. Nothing enhances our feeling of control more than by gaining power in some way. This tendency comes out in our interactions with each other; in fact, it dictates much of human relations.

Every child has significantly increased anxiety when they leave home to begin school, regardless of their family situation. They want to be accepted but there is also the greater need to diminish their fear. The need to get rid of fear and gain power is played out in forming cliques, excluding others, and overt bullying.

Researchers did a study of students who have been bullied versus the bullies to see if there was any difference in their physiological makeup.[15] They looked at the levels of a substance called C-reactive protein (CRP), which is elevated in the presence of inflammation; it's often used to determine the presence of a hidden infection. Chronically elevated levels also indicate a stressed and overactive immune system. It is not desirable to have an elevated CRP.

The study revealed that children who had been bullied had significantly elevated levels of CRP compared to those who had not been bullied. Being bullied as your introduction to the real world is not a great start. What I find even more disturbing is that the levels of CRP in bullies was lower than the norm. As it turns out, there is both a social and physiological reward for possessing more power. How all of this plays out in adulthood is not subtle. Why would you want to give up power and control? Especially when feeling the pain of anxiety is the other option.

Every child does have a strong need to be accepted, yet what should we make of the fact that it gives him or her more power (and self-esteem) to reject someone else? This is an endless loop, the root cause of which is the solvable problem of anxiety.

## Your Personal Brain Scanner

Another aspect of human consciousness exacerbates what can be a relentless barrage of negative thoughts. While we all have characteristics that allow us to thrive in our specific environment, the human body is not designed for that purpose; it is designed to survive—that is it. It is not intended to have a great time. Among our earliest ancestors, only the most anxious and alert survived. The social aspect of humans and of other higher-level mammals evolved because the species that could cooperate with one other had a higher chance of survival.

Every second of your life depends on your brain scanning your surroundings for trouble. This unconscious process guides your behavior so as to avoid danger. You will become conscious of this ongoing interaction with the environment only when a given need is unmet. This is especially true for basic survival needs such as air, food, water, excretion, sleep, and not being in pain. You will initially become nervous and then anxious. If the solution is delayed, you will become angry and your body will kick in more adrenaline and cortisol, which increases your odds of survival.

Humans additionally have consciousness so there is a secondary level of needs that can become a problem if unmet, including social interaction, self-esteem, companionship, validation, etc. It doesn't matter if your thoughts in this arena are based on reality; the default mode for your brain is negative. This characteristic causes many errors in thinking. As errors in thinking are usually irrational, there is no solution and no end. The relentless anxiety becomes unbearable and worsens with age and repetition.

We assume that solving problems will diminish our anxiety—whether it's a lawsuit, being overweight, or your chronic pain, for example. It might be true for that specific situation for a short time. But it has become obvious to me that even if I solve the respective problem, I will still experience anxiety, as my brain will continue to scan everything around me for more danger. If there is nothing physical to be concerned about then I will experience (create) endless irrational thoughts that are disruptive. In fact, when things are quiet, these thoughts often become even more intense.

One recurring example is when someone does not return an email or phone call in a timely manner. I immediately assume that I said or did something that offended the person. Or maybe they just no longer care for me. My brain immediately begins spinning. Invariably, I find out that they were out of town or dealing with a difficult situation. The delay had nothing to do with me.

A few weeks ago, I sent an email to a good friend to have re-sent out to a group of colleagues. When it was not posted I got upset. Instead of just re-sending the email or asking what happened, I spent hours obsessing about what I could have done or said that upset him. It turns out that he hadn't seen it. He happened to run across it while cleaning out his inbox and really liked it. My hours spent being agitated were a complete waste of time.

There are endless problems created by your personal scanner, which is always on high alert. Scanning the environment for danger is your body's main priority, which creates several problems.

Commonly, some of my patients are so focused on the situation or person who wronged them that it consumes their lives. Many research papers have documented the relationship between anger and increased pain. It has also been shown that people who blame their problems on other people or situations have more dysfunction and pain.[16] I've had many intense conversations with patients around this scenario. They are convinced that when their lawsuit or claim is resolved they will be happier. That is simply not true. First of all, these situations rarely resolve quickly. Meanwhile, your pain and anger pathways have become deeply imbedded and solving the problem will not reverse those circuits. What if the problem is not solvable? Do you really want to remain miserable?

Second, one problem might get solved, but is that your only one? Life constantly throws us curve balls. How many of your issues do you need to solve before you are content? What are the odds of every problem being solved to the point where you are now happy? It's not going to happen, and if it could, you would then worry when it was all going to fall apart.

Third, your brain will immediately land on another problem. Observe yourself on a day where you have some time to relax. How often does your mind take off on some issue at work or home? My first clue that this was a problem occurred when my son was about five years old. I would come home about six o'clock every evening regardless of the amount of work I still had to do and we would play catch. He was a talented pitcher and it was incredibly enjoyable getting outside with him. Unfortunately, I was also bringing home over a foot of paperwork to finish. One particularly beautiful summer evening, I was playing catch and began to notice that my mind was on my unfinished work and not enjoying my time with my family. It was not subtle and I realized that it was a common occurrence. Although it took a while to evolve, that moment of awareness helped me begin a process of letting go and engaging in the moment I was in.

Fourth, if you cannot truly relax on a given day without worrying, when are you going to regenerate? It is critical to relax when you have the opportunity. When do you get to really enjoy your life?

Your personal brain scanner cannot be turned off, otherwise you would die. Understanding this basic function of your nervous system is important and as you become aware of how this plays out on a daily basis, you can solve it.

## Descent into the Abyss—An Overview

Chronic pain is a complex neurological problem that is being more clearly understood with modern dynamic brain imaging studies. We are finding that the following areas need to be considered:

1. The source of the pain (Chapter 2)
   It may or may not be readily identifiable.
2. Sensitization (Chapter 3)
   The unconscious brain responds to repetition by recruiting more neurons.
3. Memorization (Chapter 3)
   Occurs quickly, as pain impulses fire rapidly.
4. The "modifiers" (Chapters 4 and 5)
   Sleep, anxiety, and anger each heightens the perception of pain by altering the body's chemistry.

The level of your pain is determined by your brain's interpretation of the pain signals, as well your body's chemical state. Keep in mind that mental pain and physical pain are processed in similar parts of the brain, so it's possible that a constant stream of negative thoughts are contributing to—or even the source of—your chronic pain. Understanding how you became enmeshed in this mess is the first step toward your freedom.

# CHAPTER 2

## The Source of Your Pain

LIKE ALL SURGEONS, I AM FOCUSED ON FINDING THE SOURCE of your pain so I can provide you with a solid diagnosis and surgically solve your problem. When I am successful, you are happy and I am happy. I'm the hero.

The goal is to locate the place where the pain is being generated. In my experience, it often can't be identified. Nonetheless, almost universally, surgeons tend to believe that their search will be successful, that they will find an identifiable pain source (anatomic abnormality) that they call the "pain generator." Patients also usually believe this. If the problem can be identified and repaired with surgery, the thinking goes, the pain will resolve. On the surface, this seems plausible. If you were experiencing intense back pain, for instance, you'd think there would be a diagnostic test that could identify its source and point to a solution.

It's not unlike how we think about car repair. If a part of your car is broken, you go and get it fixed. If something in your body is broken, you also go and get it fixed, right? Wrong! There is a major fallacy within this approach. Automobiles are not living creatures and therefore do not have protective pain systems. They do not possess pain fibers, a nervous system that interprets pain signals, hormones, emotions, or memories.

Acute pain is a physical link to the environment that is necessary for survival and living a functional life. It causes conscious or unconscious anxiety, a signal that you have reached the structural limits of a given body part. People without protective sensation eventually have their joints disintegrate into a "bag of bones." The resultant deformities are severe and crippling. It is most common in diabetics suffering from peripheral neuropathy and patients with leprosy. The survival for those born without pain receptors, a condition called *congenital indifference to pain* is about twelve to fifteen years. Parents can do nothing to teach these children how to protect themselves. Every attempt to replicate the pain system for those who lack one has failed. So our pain system is a wonderfully balanced, intricate, and *necessary* mechanism for survival.[1]

During my first eight years of practice, finding and repairing the "pain generator" was my main guiding principle. I assumed that if a patient had experienced low back pain for six months, then it was my role and responsibility to find the anatomic source of pain and surgically resolve it. I was diligent in this regard until I was forced to change my thinking. I finally realized that this approach was not working. Many patients experienced poor outcomes or had more pain than they had prior to their surgery. Now, I only perform surgery for structural problems, and not *all* structural problems.

The concepts in this book are applicable to any emotional or physical pain regardless of the source; but I use the spine for purposes of illustration, only because this is my area of expertise.

## Classification of Pain Sources

Dr. Howard Schubiner helped me conceptualize the following potential sources of pain.[2]

1. *Tissues (including bones, muscles, ligaments, fascia)*
   a. Structural: an anatomical abnormality identifiable on a diagnostic test with *matching* symptoms.
   b. Non-structural: a lesion resulting from conditions such as inflammation, micro-tearing, or overuse, which cannot be seen on a diagnostic test; or symptoms that do not correspond to an identified structural abnormality.
2. *Nervous System*

   Neurophysiologic disorder (NPD): causes you to experience painful symptoms whether or not you are injured. It occurs via the direct triggering of nerve pathways and/or the body's secretion of adrenaline and cortisol due to a stressful situation.

In all three of these scenarios—structural source, non-structural source, and NPD—the nervous system is rapidly bombarded by pain impulses from the body's receptors. The pain pathways, which are quickly memorized, must be considered in every patient regardless of the source of the pain.

### *Tissues—Structural Sources*

A structural abnormality is one that is distinctly identifiable on an imaging test and correlates with the patient's symptoms. A common example of a structural problem is sciatica from a pinched nerve. Each nerve in the body has a distinct corresponding pain pattern. There is often an associated numbness, weakness, or loss of a reflex.

Sciatica usually occurs in the case of a ruptured disc between the fourth and fifth lumbar vertebra pinching the fifth lumbar nerve. The typical resulting pain down the side of the leg is a perfect match. A ruptured disc between the fifth lumbar and first sacral vertebra will cause pain down the back of the leg, which is the pattern for the first sacral nerve. If in either of these two examples the pain was going down the front of the leg, it would not be considered the cause of the pain because that is the path of the fourth lumbar nerve root and it does not match.

Back pain is what we call a "non-specific complaint" and is almost always a non-structural problem. One of the few cases where it might be considered a structural problem is if there is instability between the vertebrae of more than three to four millimeters. (The distance is measured by X-rays taken with the patient bending forward as far as possible and then backward.) If the vertebrae are sliding back and forth too much, it is commonly considered to be the pain generator. I am still hesitant to perform surgery in this case since the pain could be coming from the soft tissues supporting the spine; I have not been convinced that this extra movement is a source of pain. The term for this condition is an *unstable spondylolisthesis*. Most people have some misalignment of several vertebrae without any movement. This is would be called a *stable spondylolisthesis* and would not be considered a pain source.

Destructive structural lesions such as cancer, infection, or a fracture are rare structural problems, but physicians are continuously on the lookout for the possibility.

A condition called degenerative disc disease is often cited as a structural source of chronic lower back pain (LBP). Multiple research studies, however, have shown this to be inaccurate, regardless of the severity of the degeneration.[3] (See more on this below.) In truth, physicians can identify the source of LBP only about 15 percent of the time.[4]

## Case Study: My Own Spine Surgery

Shortly after completing my orthopedic residency in 1985, I was putting my sleeping one-year old son, Nick, into his crib. Not wanting to wake him,

I was extra careful in gently reaching over the rails to lay him down. As I did this, I felt a small twinge in my left big toe. Next thing I knew, I was spending the next twelve hours flat on the floor of a friend's house with my toe screaming pain. I had ruptured my L5-S1 disc. It was a structural problem in that my left 5th nerve root was pinched and the pattern of pain was in the path of the 5th lumbar nerve root. Surgery was an option to take the pressure off this nerve. Not all structural problems require surgery, however, and I wanted to wait it out.

After sleeping no more than two to three hours a night for six weeks, I finally elected to undergo an operation that removed both the herniated disc and bone spur at L5-S1. In the meantime, I had lost twenty-five pounds, developed multiple ulcers in my stomach, and went into kidney failure.

The surgery was complicated in that the disc had ruptured into the foramen out to the side of the spine and a procedure that would normally be completed in an hour and a half took four hours. My immune system was compromised from my extreme weight loss and lack of sleep. Eleven days later, I developed a deep wound infection, which got worse when a local surgeon slashed it open in the ER. I required a second operation to wash it out. I was on intravenous antibiotics for six weeks and I could not work. I also lost my job as a spine fellow.

In addition to enduring the tribulations of being sick, I also experienced the trauma of not being able to take care of myself or my family. I will never forget how vulnerable I felt as I came to understand how little mercy there is in a capitalistic society. I had an incredibly benevolent partner who financially carried me through for a few months and I got my job back. However, this period still ranks among the darkest of my life.

The infection eventually resolved and my toe pain disappeared. The pinched L5 nerve causing my big toe to hurt was a structural problem caused by the bone spur and disc surrounding my nerve. The symptoms exactly matched the spur and indeed, they did resolve with surgery.

Until I went through this ordeal, I never understood why my spine patients complained so much. Words cannot do justice to this type of intense suffering. My entire outlook and approach to pain changed and I quickly developed a deeper understanding of the issues around back problems, including the inability to work and take care of one's family.

### Tissues—Non-Structural Sources

It was clear from the beginning of my orthopedic training that most of my patients' pains were not identifiable on a diagnostic test. This was frustrating, as I was eager to surgically solve whatever I could. My patients were even more frustrated than I was—they were the ones who suffered and wanted a rapid resolution. The possibility of providing it was a significant part of my motivation to become a surgeon.

*Non-structural pain* is where the source of pain cannot be identified on an imaging study. The distribution of the pain is usually vague and can originate from almost any structure supporting the spine, including ligaments, tendons, discs, the envelopes of tissue surrounding muscles called *fascia*, and the layers of tissue covering bones called *periosteum*. Overuse is probably the most common cause of pain, as are injuries such as sprains, strains, and tendonitis. It's often unclear what sets off inflammation. No diagnostic test can reliably identify a soft tissue problem, and yet it is much more likely to be the pain source than a structural problem.

Also note that while there may be anatomical abnormalities in your spine, if the pain doesn't match the expected patterns, they are irrelevant.

In some cases, pain patterns can mimic each other and can be hard to sort out. Some examples are:

- Thoracic 11 nerve travels to the lower abdomen and can mimic appendicitis on the right and diverticulitis on the left. One of my friends first underwent an appendectomy before his doctor realized it was a pinched T11 nerve. His pain quickly disappeared after I surgically relieved the pressure on the T11 nerve root. To make matters worse, his appendix surgery resulted in severe bleeding, which took a second operation to stop.

- Lumbar 3 nerve pain down the front of the leg can be similar to pain caused under the kneecap (*chondromalacia patella*). I have seen several patients who underwent knee arthroscopy before they realized it was a pinched L3 nerve root. An L3 decompressive surgery solves it each time.

- Lumbar 5 pain down the side of the leg can also be caused by a tendonitis of the *iliotibial band (IT)*. The IT band is a wide band of tendon that connects the pelvis to the lower leg and stabilizes your leg as you walk.

- Other problems that can light up a single nerve are *diabetic mono-neuritis*, shingles, and neurophysiologic disorder.

- Groin pain can be caused by almost any of the lumbar nerve roots but also be a symptom of *hip arthritis*. I have encountered several mistakenly performed spine surgeries when the problem was hip arthritis, and it was no surprise that they failed to resolve the pain. One patient I treated years ago had undergone four failed spine surgeries before someone realized that his symptoms were from his hip. Failing to identify hip arthritis is one of my biggest concerns, and I teach my fellows to look for it in every spine patient, making sure to include the hip in all spine X-rays.

Doctors who are able to get a thorough patient history and perform a thorough physical examination will usually have enough information to identify inflamed areas. For example, the doctor can diagnose the above-mentioned iliotibial band syndrome by putting pressure over the prominence on the side of the hip and creating pain. Patients also cannot sleep on that side. Pushing down on the kneecap and re-creating their usual pain is effective in diagnosing chondromalacia patella, which is a pain under the kneecap from softening of the cartilage.

•••••

Frequently, non-structural pain will persist over a period of months or even years. This isn't surprising when you consider that irritated tissues in any part of the body can remain inflamed almost indefinitely through normal daily activities. For example, if you sprained your ankle and kept re-spraining it daily, how long would it remain painful? On the other hand, broken bones heal in three to four months. The prognosis for a fractured spine is better than the prognosis for a muscle sprain.[5]

Patients often wonder how soft tissue lesions can be so painful. It's because soft tissues are so densely loaded with many kinds of sensory receptors, including those for light touch and pressure, position sense, hot and cold, and sharp and dull. Irritated soft tissues give rise to some of the most painful conditions, such as plantar fasciitis, tennis elbow, muscular tension headaches, chondromalacia of the kneecap, and countless more. Even a heart attack is fundamentally a muscular pain: the heart muscle lacks oxygen and the soft tissue pain fibers around it are stimulated.

One of my own muscle/tendon afflictions is *tennis elbow*. I will set it off when I lift weights that are too heavy during my workouts or I over-practice my bad golf swing. The suffering may last for months with severe pain in either one or both of my elbows. My two most severe episodes of tennis elbow lasted about eighteen months each. It hurt to shake hands, reach up and adjust the lights during surgery, use surgical instruments, or grasp anything that required grip pressure. The pain was as severe as any pain I have experienced, and it was persistent. Years after my last bout, I could still push the spot on my elbow and slightly feel the irritated area. Yet if I had an X-ray, MRI, CT scan, or bone scan of the area, the results would be completely normal.

## Degenerative Disc Disease

Degenerative disc disease is a condition in which the discs between the vertebrae lose their water content, narrow, and often collapse. As the bones of the spine move closer together and the disc dehydrates, the spine becomes less flexible. When I am required to perform surgery on a collapsed disc, they are essentially fused together and I have to use a large chisel to break them apart.

Patients often ask me if degenerated discs are a legitimate a source of back pain. My answer is always this: there is little correlation between the presence of degenerated discs and low back pain. This has been shown with X-rays, CT scans, and MRI scans. There is a lot that we don't know about the cause of low back pain, but the lack of correlation between degeneration and pain is one fact that has been consistently documented. If you take volunteers who have never experienced low back pain and obtain MRI scans, about half will have some disc degeneration by the age of fifty. By the time an asymptomatic person is sixty-five years old, the incidence of disc degeneration is around 100 percent. This also applies to bulging discs, herniated or ruptured discs, bone spurs, facet arthritis, and arthritis.[3]

You may have seen an X-ray of your spine that shows severe disc degeneration. One or more discs may have almost completely disappeared. The implication is that with the degeneration so severe, the disc must be the source of your pain, and there are many fusions performed for this problem. I feel that the collapsed disc is the least likely source of pain because there is essentially no motion. Only unstable discs can generate pain. If there is so little movement, how can they be a source of pain?

A study published in the 1950s looked at the incidence of low back pain after a simple disc excision. Interestingly, the patients with the least back pain had more arthritis on their X-ray and less motion on flexion/extension X-rays.

I see this lack of correlation between disc degeneration and pain every day I spend in clinic. I evaluate patients for sciatica and other different types of leg pains, and many of them have extensive degeneration of their spine at multiple levels. Although their leg pain can be extreme, they often (usually) have no low back pain. Conversely, I will frequently see patients with severe back pain and a completely normal MRI.

Regarding an individual degenerated disc, we do know it can go through a painful phase as it breaks down. The rings that contain the central amorphous disc material have a high density of pain fibers. This pain tends to be severe and of short duration, although even that observation is speculation. The problem with calling a given disc a structural problem is that it's not possible to tell which disc might the painful one at a specific point in time. If a person eventually ruptures an L4-5 disc, then the preceding episodes of axial low back pain were probably from that disc. However, during that period of episodic low back pain, we don't have the tools to accurately figure it out.

Several tests are used to define spine anatomy. A CAT scan and X-rays will accurately show bony anatomy well, revealing bone spurs, facet arthritis, and disc narrowing. An MRI, which looks more at the soft tissues, will show the hydration of the disc. None of these anatomic findings have been correlated with pain. A *discogram* is a procedure where an iodine dye is injected into a disc in an attempt to reproduce the patient's usual pain. It is too subjective and has fallen out of favor. None of these tests are accurate enough to justify major surgical decisions regarding non-specific LBP. Yet hundreds of thousands of spine fusions and artificial disc surgeries are performed in the U.S. every year for LBP with less than a 30 percent success rate after a two-year follow up.[6]

Many professionals feel the term "disease" should be discarded. A better term might be "progressive disc degeneration" or "normally aging spine." Degenerative disc disease is not a disease.

## Case Study: Severe Degeneration and No LBP

Joni is a fifty-something year old woman who used to be an avid cyclist and runner. She spontaneously developed extreme pain down the side of her left leg every time she stood up or walked, with no pain while sitting or lying down. She had narrowing around her fifth lumbar nerve root as it exited out of the side of her spine. Every time she stood up, the fifth nerve was tightly pinched. She had a classic structural problem.

Her spine was one of the worst looking I have ever seen in any person of any age. Every disc was completely collapsed and each vertebra was bone against bone. There was also a moderate amount of curvature called *scoliosis*. She had absolutely no back pain, which emphasizes the point that a stable spine, regardless of how bad it looks, is not a structural problem and therefore would not be considered part of the surgical decision-making discussion. I addressed the structural problem of the narrowing around the fifth lumbar nerve by removing bone around the nerve and performing a one-level fusion at L5-S1. The fusion relieved the pressure and also prevented the opening around her fifth nerve from collapsing when she stood up. Her leg pain is gone and she is back to full activities with severely degenerated discs. She is cycling and running at a pace she had prior to her pain.

I see similar cases weekly. Patients with severely degenerated spines will present with structural leg pain from a pinched nerve and no back pain. Joni's case was more extreme in the severity of the degeneration of the discs and her significant scoliosis. She still did not have LBP. If the spine is stable, whether or not it is curved, it is not considered a structural problem, so it is an unlikely source of pain.

### Central Nervous System—Neurophysiologic Disorder (NPD)

When you are under stress for any reason, all of the fifty trillion cells[7] in your body are bathed in adrenaline, cortisol and other stress chemicals, and each organ system will react in its own unique way. Consequently, there are over thirty physical manifestations of this situation. There have been several terms used to describe this problem. I feel the most accurate description is neurophysiologic disorder.

Dr. Howard Schubiner is a leading authority on NPD, and his preferred term for this diagnosis is *mind-body syndrome (MBS)*. Others include:

- Tension myositis syndrome (TMS)[8]
- Central sensitization syndrome (CSS)
- Psychophysiological disorder (PPD)
- Stress illness syndrome
- Psychosomatic disorder

All of these diagnoses describe the same phenomenon: your body's over-reactive response to sustained sensory input. Here are thirty-three symptoms that Dr. Schubiner lists in his book, *Unlearn Your Pain.*[2]

1. Heartburn, acid reflux
2. Abdominal pains
3. Irritable bowel syndrome
4. Tension headaches
5. Migraine headaches
6. Unexplained rashes
7. Anxiety and/or panic attacks
8. Depression

9. Obsessive-compulsive thought patterns

10. Eating disorders

11. Insomnia

12. Fibromyalgia

13. Back pain

14. Neck pain

15. Shoulder pain

16. Repetitive stress injury

17. Carpal tunnel syndrome

18. Reflex sympathetic dystrophy (RSD)

19. Temporomandibular joint syndrome (TMJ)

20. Chronic tendonitis

21. Facial pain

22. Numbness, tingling sensations

23. Fatigue or chronic fatigue syndrome

24. Palpitations

25. Chest pain

26. Hyperventilation

27. Interstitial cystitis/spastic bladder (irritable bladder syndrome)

28. Pelvic pain

29. Muscle tenderness

30. Postural orthostatic tachycardia (POTS)

31. Tinnitus

32. Dizziness

33. Post Traumatic Stress Disorder (PTSD)

## Triggers

Your nervous system has a sustained chemical response to unrelenting thoughts or other sensations, and it can also create symptoms based on prior traumas. The term for this is "triggering." If you encounter a situation that resembles a prior traumatic one, your body will respond the same way it did when the first incident occurred. Why would you have the same symptoms? *Because the neural pain pathways that developed when you were first traumatized are permanent and can be reactivated.* For example, let's suppose you were bullied in fifth grade by a classmate who was taller with fair skin and blonde hair. He wore glasses and had an unusually high-pitched voice. Imagine that as an adult, you inadvertently cut in front of someone at the checkout counter and a person bearing a resemblance to your childhood bully spoke harshly to you. Your brain would hear a voice and see a visual profile just like the bully's. Even though, intellectually, you would know that this was a different person, you might have an automatic and strong response, quickly feeling anxious and upset. The incident might even set off a chain of unpleasant physical reactions, including perspiring, your heart skipping, and shortness of breath from your body's release of adrenaline and cortisol.

I frequently see patients who've had a successful surgery but later return to my office with a recurrence of the same symptoms they experienced pre-surgery. I occasionally repeat the diagnostic testing, but most of the time I don't find a cause for the flare-up. Now I wait a few weeks to order the tests; if some circumstance or particular stress has stimulated the old pain pathway (which is often the case), re-implementing the reprogramming tools will calm down the pain within a couple of days.

Dr. Schubiner tells the story of a physician whose left leg was crushed when his helicopter was shot down in the Vietnam War.[2] Multiple surgeries later, he had an almost normally functioning leg. Several times a year, however, he would experience severe pain and swelling in his leg, lasting several days and sometimes up to a week. During these periods, he was quite incapacitated, but afterward his leg would return to normal. Every test for a new injury would come out negative.

His symptoms suddenly returned one day while he was walking with his wife in a park and almost fell to the ground. His wife looked at him and asked, "Did you hear the helicopter?" "No," he replied. His brain, however, *had* heard it.

While this man's situation might seem like a psychological issue, it's not. He wasn't imagining his symptoms. Rather, the symptoms were linked to pain pathways that were triggered by his brain and nervous system. His initial injury had occurred while helicopters were flying overhead in Vietnam (the unique set of circumstances). When he encountered similar circumstances, even if he didn't consciously recognize them, the memory/pain pathways were re-stimulated.

## The Light Switch

A trigger for pain pathways can be compared to a light switch. When you flip the switch, the switch doesn't turn on; instead, it's the light bulb that's usually at least several feet away, connected by wiring. Likewise, if the "pain switch" in your brain that connects to your knee is on, it is your knee that will hurt, not your brain.

It's still a challenging concept to understand, but here is a story that shows how it works: One Labor Day my wife and I were looking for a used car. At one dealership, we got into a car to see how it felt. As I climbed out of it, I suddenly felt extreme pain over my right sacroiliac joint. It was indescribably sharp and, of course, everyone at the dealership was concerned and offered me all types of help. I was worried and unsure what had caused it to happen.

In the moment, I had no idea what had happened, but later that afternoon, I realized that I'd been triggered by a lively (heated) discussion with my wife about what type of car to purchase. The trigger was a result of my post-traumatic stress disorder (PTSD) reaction (NPD) following my two back surgeries that included multiple complications. I also hadn't been practicing the tools to calm down my nervous system, which will be discussed later in this book. Within a day of re-engaging in the tools (and an apology), I was free of the pain. What was fascinating to me was that when I pushed on my back it was painful directly where I touched it. Because of this, I thought it was a structural issue, and initially did not classify it as NPD.

## Other NPD Considerations

In addition to the direct physical symptoms created by an adverse chemical makeup, NPD has the indirect effect of causing you to neglect your health. Being trapped by so many unpleasant symptoms is miserable, and chances are you will become frustrated and angry. Anger is always destructive, including self-destructive. You simply don't care. Why else would you allow yourself to evolve into such terrible physical shape? I feel it is akin to a "slow suicide."

Another consideration is the barrier that NPD presents to participating in the healing process. One common NPD symptom is having irrational obsessive thought patterns, which do not respond to reason. You can become focused on being "fixed," think that "the doctor is missing something," or "there must be something wrong." There is something wrong in that your body's nervous system and chemistry are seriously out of balance. The first step is to understand how to solve this problem. I have learned that these adrenalized neurological circuits can block one's willingness to learn. When I encounter this situation with a patient, there is no persuading them—I have to let go.

One of the most serious problems that is created by untreated NPD is the effect it has on others, specifically anger-fueled NPD. It's no wonder that chronic pain patients are angry; it's a condition that creates an indescribable depth of frustration. But it has a terrible effect on those around you: when you are angry, it is all about you. You lose awareness of the needs of others, and lack of awareness is the essence of abuse. Spouses and children of patients in chronic pain become the targets of this deep anger, and the cycle of adverse childhood events continues. There is a high chance that these children will act out their frustrations at school. Also, their parents have modeled anger as the normal way of dealing with adversity.

## My Struggle with NPD

I've probably had NPD since elementary school but did not experience any extreme symptoms until my descent into a burnout during my spinal deformity fellowship in 1985. Initially, I didn't realize I was headed into a downward spiral; I felt light-headed a couple of times and had to scrub out of surgery, but I just blamed it on not having a good breakfast. Then, four years later, I had a panic attack while driving across a bridge late at night. I had no idea what was going on, as I still was not emotionally experiencing anything that I would have labeled as anxiety. My identity was that of a fearless spine surgeon, and I was. My body was telling me something very different, however. By 1996, I was experiencing sixteen of the thirty-three above-mentioned NPD[2] symptoms and no one, even after diagnostic testing, had a clue as to the cause.

My symptoms were:

1. Migraine headaches
2. Migratory skin rashes
3. Burning in both feet
4. Obsessive-compulsive disorder (OCD)
5. Post-traumatic stress disorder (PTSD)
6. Anxiety reactions/panic attacks
7. Heartburn/acid reflux
8. Tinnitus
9. Depression

10. Chronic tendonitis
11. Insomnia
12. Neck/low back pain
13. Chest pain
14. Heart palpitations
15. Tension headaches
16. Itching on my scalp

My obsessive-compulsive disorder was an "internal" form of OCD with intrusive thoughts that were constantly battling with counter-thoughts. The prognosis for OCD is dismal and I almost didn't make it through this ordeal. My downward spiral was complete and I did not have any hope. I can look any patient in the eye and say, "You may be suffering as much as I did but not more."

I didn't learn any of these concepts in my medical training; instead, I experimented with many different methods before I found a combination of tools that worked best for me. By 2004, all of my NPD symptoms had resolved and I was not only back on my feet but able to thrive. My wife has reminded me, however, that when I stop using the tools, my symptoms will begin to return in about two to three weeks. My pain circuits are permanent and can be reawakened.

## My Migraines

To help you understand how and when NPD symptoms can develop, I will rewind here and explain how mine started.

I was five years old and living with my family in a small town in New Hampshire. Our house was directly across the street from the town common. We heard that the Fourth of July fireworks were going to be launched in the common, just a few hundred feet of our front door. I was excited and I counted down the weeks until the big event.

The Fourth finally arrived, and around 4 p.m. that day I developed a headache. I didn't remember ever having one this severe and within an hour it had progressed into a piercing migraine. That evening, the fireworks began at 10 p.m. For almost an hour the house was rocked with explosions that were dramatically magnified in my pulsating brain. I don't have the words to describe the unpleasantness of the evening. The only good news was that my usually raging mother stopped to put a cold washcloth on my head. Throughout my upbringing, the severity of my migraines was one event that would always bring a dead halt to her screaming.

This festive event marked the beginning of a lifetime of migraine headaches. I would develop a severe headache every two or three weeks that usually was associated with projectile vomiting. I used to welcome that phase in that my headache would abate a little, after the vomiting. I would be stuck in bed motionless for eight to twelve hours. Every movement was excruciating. I don't know if I would ever fall asleep, as I seemed to drift in and out of consciousness. I was always fine the next morning, but I could never tell what might set the next one off.

In the 1980s, a migraine drug called Imitrex was developed. It was administered by injection, and if I could inject my thigh in time, the migraine would be cut short or avoided. That medication had a huge impact on my life. The only problem was that, since it was an injectable, I would frequently wait a little too long before using it.

Migraines are nasty and I didn't know it was an NPD symptom until I was introduced to the diagnosis in 2011 by Dr. Schubiner. In looking back on my childhood, I realize that my headaches were a stress-related response to my mother's rage (more on this later in the book). I no longer have migraine headaches and quit buying the drugs years ago. If I get a sense one might be occurring, a little coffee and Ibuprofen knocks it right down.

## The Source of Your Pain—Final Thoughts

I frequently compare surgery to dental work. Generally, a dentist can identify a painful structural problem, such a cavity that has gone down to the root. In that case, your dentist can solve the problem with a filling, root canal, crown, extraction, etc. But what if your diagnosis was "mouth pain" without an identifiable source? It could be a sinus infection, gum disease, or a symptom of NPD such as temporomandibular joint dysfunction (TMJ). If your dentist proceeds to operate on one of your teeth without a firm diagnosis, it's unlikely that he or she will solve your problem. You can only fix what you can see, and surgery should be performed as a last resort only when everything else has been tried.

The principles presented in this chapter apply to any and all areas of your body, not just to your spine. This includes every organ system, the only difference being the methods you will use to make the correct diagnosis. Whether or not you have a structural problem, addressing all aspects of your pain experience is your best chance of resolving it.

# CHAPTER 3

# Imbedding Pain Pathways

WE'VE SEEN HOW EMOTIONAL AND PHYSICAL PAIN impulses can become permanently imbedded into our nervous systems. As the weeks and months go by and the impulses are repeated over and over, profound chemical and neurological changes take place. This chapter discusses the neurological changes of sensitization and memorization, which dramatically alter our perception of pain.

The brain works by association, so pain quickly becomes connected to the situation that caused it. We learn what to do to avoid danger, and then we do it each time we re-encounter that danger. It only takes one time for us to put a hand too close to the flame, feeling the heat, and realizing it can burn us to keep us from intentionally doing it again. Our brain, though, with what is called the *nociceptive system*, automatically guides our behavior to avoid pain and remain safe. Although you probably don't realize it, when you are sitting on a chair, your body is constantly shifting to avoid damage to your skin. If you feel pain, that means your body has exceeded the pain threshold. This protective mechanism does not exist in people who are completely paralyzed, so pressure sores may occur from skin breakdown. Most of the time, we are not aware of the incredible benefits of our pain avoidance system.

However, this same mechanism of deeply remembered associations does not always serve us as well for emotional pain. We assess our environment for risk and opportunity as part of our sensory input. We avoid people who do not speak nicely to us. We look for meaningful social interactions and connection with others. However, our mind also creates risks that are not real. The term for this phenomenon is *cognitive distortions.* Examples include labeling ourselves and others, "should" thinking, mind reading, and emotional reasoning. Another descriptive term is "fast thinking" as opposed to rational or "slow thinking."[1] Humans jump to conclusions based on their own past experience, without analyzing all the data all of the time. Often these assumptions tend to be negative and inaccurate. When they are repeated quickly and frequently enough they may become programmed into our brains as our reality. But it is reality only from our individual perspective. Unfortunately, when our brains process these negative assumptions, the body's protective chemical reactions are the same as if it were responding to physical pain. The stress reactions become sustained and are extremely unpleasant over time.

## Pain Sensitization

When the brain is hammered with unpleasant emotional or physical impulses day after day, week after week, it becomes more and more efficient in processing them. Subsequently, it takes less of an impulse to elicit the same response in the brain. It's this process, called sensitization, that causes patients to complain that their pain is getting much worse in spite of the lack of additional trauma.

The sensitization phenomenon was documented in a 2004 clinical research study in which volunteers who had no significant experience with chronic pain had a carefully measured pressure stimulus applied to their thumbs.[2] The response was measured in the brain with a functional MRI (fMRI), which is able to track metabolic activity. Researchers consistently identified one small area of the brain that responded to the stimulus. Next, they applied the same stimulus to patients who'd had chronic pain for more than three months. In this second group, five parts of the brain lit up; their pain response was much greater. The difference in intensity of the response was consistent and dramatic.

Water torture provides a crude example of how the brain gets sensitized. In this scenario, a prisoner is strapped to a board and water is dripped on his forehead. The intensity of the drip remains the same, but because of the repetition, the nervous system becomes focused on the dripping and the sensation becomes intolerable. The victim usually goes insane. Granted, there are the added elements of fear and of being trapped, but don't people in chronic pain experience these emotions as well?

A less extreme example of pain sensitization happened to a friend of mine, Dennis, while working on a construction site. One day on the job, Dennis placed his hand on the handle of an electric masonry saw, a tool that requires a small pump to run water over the blade. At the start of the job in the morning, he felt a very mild tingling sensation when he touched the handle. As the day went on the sensation gradually became stronger. By early afternoon, the tingling was so strong that it felt like an actual shock and he could no longer bring himself to touch the handle.

The two other men on Dennis's crew gave him a hard time about it at first. They'd watched him get more and more cautious, yet when they touched the handle they could barely feel a thing.

The next day they rotated tasks, and one of the other guys worked with the saw. Initially he felt only the smallest amount of tingling, just like Dennis, but by mid-afternoon the sensation was intense and he wouldn't touch the handle, either. The third guy now thought they were playing with him. When he rotated in and first touched the handle, he couldn't feel a thing. But eventually he also wouldn't go near it; he'd become a believer. Finally, they discovered the culprit: a frayed wire. It was fixed on the fourth day.

What's interesting to me about this story is the degree of the difference in sensation over just six to seven hours of repeated exposure. If the initial sensation from the saw had been strong, the story would have seemed more plausible. However, even though the level of the electric current remained the same, it went from being barely perceptible to feeling like an electric shock. Dennis said that even the anticipation of touching the handle became a problem.

The pressure stimulus study, the water torture example, and Dennis's saw handle experience demonstrate how the central nervous system becomes more sensitized as the same stimulus recruits more neurons in the brain to fire. In each case, the pain increases with repetition. Of course, you also experience pain when you are injured and actual pain receptors are stimulated, such as when you get a bad cut or scrape. But whether it's a cut or a sensitized nervous system, the bottom line is that you feel the pain. The extent of it depends on the number of neurons firing in your brain. It's quite literally "in your head."

## Memorization of Neurological Circuits

In learning about chronic pain and how it works, it's important to distinguish it from acute pain. Acute pain is a sensation that creates a neurological response that prompts your body to try and avoid whatever caused the pain. It is present as long as the offending stimulus is there and hopefully lasts for only a few seconds or several minutes, such as when you get a bruise. It can also last for days or weeks until damaged or inflamed tissues heal, such as in the case of a broken bone. Chronic pain is pain that lasts longer than the time that's expected for the injured tissues to heal.

It has been demonstrated that chronic pain and acute pain exist in different parts of your brain. A study published in 2013[3] looked at functional MRIs of people who had been experiencing low back pain (LBP) for less than two months (subacute) and compared them to scans of patients who had been suffering for more than ten years (chronic). The subacute group showed brain activity in the known low back pain centers; while in the chronic group, the activity had unexpectedly shifted to the emotional centers. In the second part of the study, fMRI scans were done every three months in a subset of the subacute group for one year. The pain resolved in about half the volunteers but the rest of them developed chronic LBP. The brain activity shifted to the emotional area of the brain in all those who became chronic; the low back pain center became dormant. They still felt the same kind of pain, but the "driver" of the pain was completely different. This study demonstrated that chronic pain is driven by the emotional centers of the brain, rather than the pain centers.

This phenomenon might partly explain why neurological connections associated with pain often continue to function even if the offending stimulus is removed. A classic example of this is phantom limb pain. Phantom limb pain occurs in patients who require an amputation, usually because blood supply to the limb has been compromised by vascular disease such as diabetes or atherosclerosis. Prior to the amputation, lack of oxygen causes the limb to become very painful. After the limb is removed, up to 60 percent of patients feel the pain as though the limb were still there. Almost 40 percent of sufferers characterize the pain as anywhere from distressing to even more severe than before.[4]

There is not a more definitive operation than removing the entire source of pain by performing an amputation, yet the patient often feels the same sensations and pain as they did when the limb was attached.

This is a dramatic example of the power of the nervous system and a reminder that the brain is an extremely complex, sophisticated organ that can be programmed.

### Pain Pathways

To understand the development of chronic pain, it's helpful to look at the concepts in the book *The Talent Code* by Dan Coyle[5]. *The Talent Code* focuses on the idea that our most basic method of learning any skill is repetition. Coyle explains that the three aspects of creating talent in any skill are: 1) deep learning; 2) ignition (obsessive repetitions); and 3) master coaching. Within this paradigm, your brain is processing specific impulses within a narrow range to focus on learning a skill, whether it's piano, soccer, or math.

Consider the repetitions required to become a world-class virtuoso pianist. It requires years of rigorous and prolonged daily practice to attain that status and maintain it. With just a small decrease in practice time the level of performance will diminish. This type of skill is often described as "muscle memory." Of course, your muscles don't actually *learn* anything; rather, it's the laying down of neurological pathways and reinforcing them that leads the muscles to do the same thing over and over, and get better and more efficient at it. Some may say that genius is born, but in reality, it occurs after 10,000 hours of repetition.[5]

Coyle also links this process to the production of *myelin* in the nervous system. Myelin is a substance that coats nerve cells and improves conduction of impulses, similar to what insulation does for an electric wire. The more repetition, the thicker the myelin, and the faster the impulses.

Unfortunately, chronic pain fits this profile. The impulses are specific (you have already "deeply learned" them); they come in rapidly and are sustained (this is the ignition part); and since there is little variation in the pain, you don't need master coaching. This is one of the reasons chronic pain always worsens over time (usually without further injury)—your body becomes more "skilled" at processing it.

Skill pathways and pain pathways both become imbedded, but they do so at different paces. It usually takes years for a pianist's impulses to the brain to become deeply imbedded. But pain impulses are fired so rapidly—I compare it to a machine gun—that they become permanent within a matter of months.

The pain pathways become imbedded, and it's worsened by the many negative thoughts (which are also being imbedded) associated with the pain experience. It's hard to avoid becoming demoralized. Months go by, your pain won't go away, and no one seems to know why. You can't help but create stories about your pain, which evolve into memorized circuits as well.

"The surgeon screwed up my back." "I can't get out of bed." "My pain is ruining my life." These neurological circuits can take on a life of their own, running on a constant loop. If left unchecked, they may turn into a serious obstacle to recovery, one that's not a psychological issue as much as a "programming" issue. (More on this in upcoming chapters.) You become programmed to think the same thoughts over and over again. The good news is, you can develop tools to break the cycle of negative thinking, a process I call "reprogramming." It's much different from the traditional psychological approach to pain.

Remember that repetitive negative thoughts, just like physical pain impulses, are also sensory input. Like the body's response to physical pain, they also cause a protective chemical reaction to occur in addition to the body's response to physical pain. Between the two, your nervous system becomes really fired up.

### *Feeding Repetitive Negative Thoughts*

We learn many ways to deal with repetitive negative thoughts, but most of them are ineffective over the long term. Instead of getting rid of the thoughts, these methods only feed them. Think of these common coping mechanisms in terms of how they affect the neurological pathways in the brain:

1. Suffering
2. Suppressing
3. Masking

## Suffering

When you suffer, you think the same set of thoughts over and over, a process that clearly reinforces a neurological circuit. Suffering takes many forms—complaining, arguing, manipulation, gossiping, etc. You keep thinking about the mess that your life has become. The resulting anger is the jet fuel that gets these circuits really spinning. It's almost impossible to "let it go" because the anger feels so justified. Remember, I haven't even added in the perception of physical pain.

Recently, I had a patient who was convinced that his orthopedic surgeon had done a poor job on his rotator cuff surgery five years earlier. He continued to rant about how he'd been irreversibly damaged by this surgeon. (I don't know how well the surgery went or how much the patient had engaged in rehab after the surgery.) He was so focused on the story and the sensations around his shoulder that I couldn't even touch the skin around his shoulder girdle. Regardless of the reason for his condition, his daily quality of life was additionally compromised by these repetitive, ruminating thoughts.

It is common for patients in chronic pain to endlessly discuss their pain and medical care with their family and friends. Unfortunately, this greatly reinforces both the pain and negative thought pathways. Additionally, studies have consistently shown that keeping a pain diary actually delays recovery from an injury.[6] Your brain will develop wherever you place its attention, and any energy spent tracking or discussing your troubles is counter-productive.

When I first wrote this book five years ago I had a vague sense that people suffering from chronic pain spent a lot of time complaining about their pain-related problems to anyone who would listen, but I didn't realize the depth and extent of it. Now I am aware that many, if not most people in pain, spend the majority of their time complaining. I discovered this pattern during a workshop that I held at the Omega Institute in New York. One of the ground rules for the five-day course was that the participants could not discuss their pain with anyone. It initially threw them off, but by the end of the week, many of them saw that not complaining had been a significant factor in the healing process.

## Suppressing

The second strategy we use to deal with negative thoughts is to suppress them. We don't want to feel negative, so we don't. Thinking that we have no alternative to a difficult situation, we put our heads down and just move on.

I have witnessed the downside of this kind of suppressing firsthand in the medical profession. In medicine, suppression is a way of life—it's the way we "succeed." We experience extreme training conditions, famously long hours, and harsh demands. Complaining is not an option; however, the price in terms of mental health is high.

The rate of physician burnout is around 40–50 percent and has climbed almost 10 percent in the last five years.[7] There is a higher prevalence of psychiatric disorders, drug abuse, and alcoholism among physicians than in the general population.[8] The suicide rate for male physicians is

40 percent higher than in men in general; for women doctors, it's 130 percent higher than among their non-medical peers.[9] Four out of eighty of my medical school classmates and two of my close spine surgeon colleagues committed suicide. The most recent of these was a close friend who assisted me in two surgery cases on his last day. Each case had gone extremely well, after which he shook my hand and said, "Nice case." The next day he was gone.

I had watched this friend slowly fold under the stress of being a spine surgeon over the years. He suffered the deadly combination of suppressed anxiety and extreme perfectionism, and burnout was a constant threat. At the time of his death, however, he appeared to have finally gotten a handle on his issues and seemed to be on the right track. None of us saw it coming.

Trying to suppress or not think negative thoughts may even be more damaging than suffering. The more you try to ignore a negative thought, the stronger it is when it reoccurs. It also takes a significant amount of mental and emotional energy to keep such thoughts under wraps.

For example, imagine that you were upset at your spouse, partner, or child because they routinely don't pick up after themselves. You don't want to rock the boat, so you don't bring it up. As close as you are to this person, you don't want to feel frustrated. So you aren't—instead, you suppress your emotions as you try to ignore the untidiness.

Your rational brain kicks in and starts to keep score. You rationalize that this isn't that big a deal, but you are now expending a lot of mental energy. You know the rest of the story. The longer you try to ignore the problem and "think positive," the higher the chance that when you finally decide to deal with it, your eventual reaction may be irrational and disproportionate to the circumstances. Any time you are anxious or angry, your brain is in survival mode, and it's impossible to get out of it by rational means.

There has been a movement for decades that encourages people to think positive. In my opinion, this philosophy represents a sophisticated form of suppressing. If a situation is bad, it's bad. Pretending otherwise does not help. The energy spent suppressing the negative emotions could be better spent solving the problem. We will discuss this concept in more detail, but recent research shows that you have to fully embrace and feel your negativity in order to work through it. One term for this is "leaning into the negative."[14] It's important not to take verbal or physical action when you are feeling these strong emotions, but suppressing them can become disastrous. Once you've acknowledged your negativity, you can substitute a more appropriate response. This is a more positive approach than simple positive thinking.

In the above scenario, I would suggest using expressive writing and active meditation as tools to process your feelings *before* you react. It's sometimes hard not to react in the moment, but it can be done with practice and awareness. I assume that you want to maintain a loving bond with those who are close to you. Reactively firing away at them does not help nurture relationships.

*White Bears*

One research study conducted in 1987 sheds a fascinating light on what happens when we try to suppress our thoughts. The study was outlined in a paper titled, "The Paradoxical Effects of Thought Suppression," written by Dr. Daniel Wegner, a Harvard psychologist.[10] The experiment he devised is commonly referred to as "White Bears." Volunteers were divided into two groups and instructed to verbalize all their thoughts during a five-minute period in a stream of consciousness exercise. During the exercise, they were told either to think of a white bear or not think of a white bear, depending on which group they were in. Every time they had a "white bear" thought they either rang a bell or verbalized it. This is how the experimental treatments differed for the two groups:

- One group was first told to not think about white bears for five minutes. Then they were told to do the opposite: spend the next five minutes trying to think about white bears, all while engaging in the stream of consciousness exercises.
- The other group was initially instructed to think about white bears and then to not think about them during the second five minutes, while also continuing the stream of consciousness exercises.

The results were as follows:

- In both groups the participants could diminish the frequency of white bear thoughts when asked to suppress them, but no one could completely get rid of these thoughts.
- In the expression part of the experiment (where volunteers were instructed to think about white bears), the number of white bear thoughts was higher in both groups. The incidence of white bear thoughts actually increased over the five-minute span of expression.
- In the group that was initially asked to suppress the white bear thoughts there was a dramatic increase in the white bear thoughts during the expression phase compared to the group who was asked to think about white bears first.

Wegner's experiment demonstrated that trying not to think about something will markedly increase the chances of your thinking about it. There is a rebound or trampoline effect. When asked not to think about something, "not thinking" becomes associated with many other cues. In other words, imagine that you experienced a disturbing thought while attending the opera. There's a high chance that the thought would recur the next time you walked into the same building, and, as it's an unpleasant thought, you would suppress it. Then imagine the thought becomes connected to turning off a specific freeway exit or walking into the front door of your house. Now you are sweeping the thought under the rug multiple times a day. You are spending a significant amount of conscious energy on a thought that doesn't represent who you are; otherwise you wouldn't be suppressing it. Twenty years later these thoughts could become your "demons." How? They are just irrational circuits that are now parasites in your brain. The more you think about them, the stronger they will become, and they become even more of a problem if you suppress them. As dismal as this scenario sounds, it's a solvable problem.

The White Bears experiment is key to the whole mental health aspect of chronic pain. There is a lot of anxiety and frustration in the chronic pain experience and also a lot of terrible thoughts. These thoughts are usually so disturbing that we feel we have to suppress them. But in suppressing them, you are giving them power, and it will eventually take a tremendous amount of emotional and intellectual energy to ignore them. This is energy you need in order to be creative in solving your problems.

There are many research papers about the consequences of thought suppression. One paper demonstrated that it may be a key link between depression and becoming addicted to opioids.[11] In depression there is an overwhelming number of negative thoughts; what do you do with them? I did not have a choice in experiencing them; and the harder I suppressed them, the stronger they became. In retrospect, it was the factor that precip-itated my descent into obsessive-compulsive disorder (OCD), manifested by relentless intrusive thoughts.

Another disturbing paper showed that suppressing thoughts causes damage to the brain's hippocampus. This is the area that processes both short- and long-term memory.[12] It is well-documented that your brain physically shrinks in the presence of chronic pain but fortunately re-expands with its resolution.[13] You can't control your thoughts or emotions without experiencing both physical and mental consequences.

*Boys Don't Cry*

Men do not usually share their feelings the way most women do. Years ago, I began to notice the toll this was taking on my male patients. The more "manly" the man, the bigger the problem.

I had one patient, Roy, a member of a SWAT team, who had leg pain. I performed a successful surgery on him that nicely resolved his problem. About four years later, he returned with back pain and a recurrence of his leg symptoms. I knew how well the surgery had gone and thought it was unlikely that he had developed a new problem. He was also incredibly physically fit and careful with his back.

I offered to re-do Roy's MRI scan but suggested that he first re-engage in the tools I had prescribed for calming down his nervous system, which he had dropped. I was planning to reorder an MRI on his next visit. Much to my surprise, when he came back, his symptoms were gone. I decided to dig a little deeper.

I learned that Roy had been experiencing severe anxiety and there was no one he felt he could talk to, given his position. No one wants to think a SWAT team member has anxiety. The paradox is that, by simply admitting he had anxiety, and engaging in some simple somatic exercises, the level of anxiety quickly plummeted, along with that of his leg pain.

Every human being, regardless of position or role, has anxiety. In fact, the more prominent the role, the more stress, the more anxiety.

Many of us spend a tremendous amount of energy putting on the façade of being bulletproof. But none of us is, and the consequences of suppressing anxiety are high.

Pain pathways are permanent, and many situations can reactivate them. The situation can range from a highly stressful event to a trigger that the person may not even find particularly unpleasant. Recurrent symptoms often are a result of reactivating a prior pain pathway, and the intensity of pain is similar to the original ordeal. I have learned to wait a couple of weeks before reordering new diagnostic tests, unless a patient presents a compelling set of new symptoms.

## Masking

Masking your reaction to stress is a third way of dealing with repetitive negative thoughts. Masking is behavior that's used to cover up uncomfortable emotions, where you do something to get your mind off of a negative situation. Although it may be effective in the short-term, it's not sustainable. Categories of masking include:

- Addictions
  - Chemical
    - Prescription or illicit drugs
    - Alcohol
    - Cigarettes
  - Work
  - Sex
  - Gambling
  - Over-eating
- Getting caught up in a "good cause" (The cause might be excellent, but the driving force behind it could be suspect if carefully examined.)

- Hoarding
- Excessive involvement in hobbies
  - Gardening
  - Reading
  - Sports
- Extreme belief systems

Some of the activities listed above, such as hobbies, are not problematic if practiced for the right reasons. If you pursue a deep passion on your own terms and in harmony with your value system, you are creating alternate neurologic pathways that can improve your mental health. It's an important strategy in neurological reprogramming. However, following your passion is a different process than obsessively pursuing activities to outrun your anxiety.

Here's one instance where a hobby may be unhealthy: a close friend, in in his mid-eighties, reads about six to eight hours a day. On the surface it doesn't seem like much of a problem—at that age, why not? However, his reading was interfering with doing other important things. For instance, he would like to be more active but says he is too busy to regularly exercise. He has slowly realized that his reading might be obsessive. He still has not pulled out of it but he does have some awareness of the problem.

Masking strategies, even when anxiety driven, might be slightly more effective than suffering or suppressing in that they are not directly feeding the negative circuits. But, they are not slowing them down, either. When you are finished with that particular activity, the repetitive negative thoughts remain. What's more, if you have some type of chemical addiction, there are often physical and social consequences to masking.

## Imbedding Pain Pathways—Final Thoughts

The first two strategies for dealing with unpleasant thoughts—suffering and suppressing—don't work. If you're continually suffering with your mental and/or physical pain, these circuits will be reinforced. If you're trying to suppress, those repressed circuits can grow to become monsters. It's impossible to avoid thinking about your mental or physical pain for any sustained length of time. Masking pain-related thoughts might work for a short time, but the pain and distress will still be there after the masking activity is over. You will become increasingly angry and frustrated, eventually finding that you don't have the energy to continue to distract yourself, even for short periods of time. Then pain consumes your life.

Take a few minutes to consider how you use the strategies of suffering, suppressing, and masking. We all do. Suffering is easy and seductive; playing the victim can feel powerful. Complaining and gossiping makes for easy conversation. We suppress whatever makes us uncomfortable; you might have been taught to just buck up and be strong. Think about how these coping methods may be preventing you from having a deep, connected, joyous quality of life. We'll talk about healthier ways to break patterns of negative thinking in the upcoming chapters.

# CHAPTER 4

# The Modifiers—Sleep and Anxiety

WE'VE ESTABLISHED THAT PAIN COULD originate from a structural or non-structural tissue problem, or it may be a manifestation of neurophysiologic disorder (NPD). Over time, the nervous system becomes sensitized to these mental and physical pain impulses; and, eventually, these circuits are memorized.

This sequence is intertwined with another series of events I call "the modifiers," which are sleep, anxiety, and anger. The modifiers heighten your physiological response to unrelenting pain. Patients in chronic pain understandably become anxious, frustrated, and angry; their stress levels rise and they lose sleep.

Pain modifiers are important to understand because under stress, your body chemistry changes. Your stress hormones, including cortisol and adrenaline, rise. Adrenaline is the "fight or flight" hormone; when secreted, it increases heart rate, elevates blood pressure, expands the lung airways, causes perspiration, and creates many other defensive bodily responses, as described in Chapter 1. Cortisol's effect is more lasting. It maintains a state of body alertness to fend off threats. The net effect is that your pain receptors and nervous system now exist in a different chemical environment even though there's no additional physical injury, or perhaps none to begin with. What's the ultimate result? All your senses are on high alert and you will experience even more pain. Animal studies have shown that stress increases the conductivity of the peripheral nerves by 30 to 40 percent.[1]

Since adrenaline diminishes the blood supply to the frontal lobes (thinking centers), your decision-making skills are also affected. That's why it's crucial to calm down your central nervous system before making a surgical decision, where there is no turning back.

The modifiers that we'll discuss in this chapter are sleep and anxiety. Anger will be presented in Chapter 5.

## Sleep

You cannot and will not improve your quality of life without consistently sleeping seven to eight hours a night. Lack of sleep is an absolute block to recovering from chronic pain.

Sleep is so important, and yet many of us don't get enough of it. In fact, statistics tell us that over 40 percent of Americans don't get adequate sleep.[2] A common belief is that adults don't need as much sleep as children, but this is untrue. Unfortunately, people can get so used to sleeping only five to six hours a night that they feel its "normal." It's not.

The problem is worse in people suffering from chronic pain. Over 40 percent of those in this group consistently fail to get a full night's sleep, which is double that of the rest of the population.[3] Pain is often felt more keenly at night, when there are fewer distractions.

One study assessed the quality of Stage V (REM) sleep in female volunteers. REM stands for "rapid eye movement," and it is the dreaming stage. The subjects with less (and poorer quality) REM sleep had a higher sensitivity to pain.[4]

Multiple studies have correlated poor sleep with increased pain and diminished function. Lack of sleep alters perception of pain and also one's capacity to cope. It actually has a greater impact on creating disability than the severity of pain. This was rather surprising to me since I had spent my career addressing pain and never perceived sleep as a major issue. The study also showed that inadequate sleep had a greater impact on disability than leg pain. Surgeons are generally focused on sciatica and assume that treating it will resolve their patient's problems.[5]

What was even more surprising to me was that I had always assumed patients in pain could not sleep because of their pain. It's actually the opposite scenario. A large, four-year study in Israel showed that it was lack of sleep that induced chronic pain, and not the other way around. A patient who has insomnia has more than a 40 percent higher chance of experiencing chronic pain.[6]

When I began to address sleep with my patients, I felt I had found a whole, simple and effective new weapon. I was surprised at how much better my patients felt with improved sleep, and how quickly they improved. Their pain decreased, and there was a marked improvement in their sense of well-being. Occasionally, just improving sleep alone (without the other tools in my structured care program), would relieve the pain. Most patients initially require sleep medications for three to six months while getting past their pain. It is easier to decrease their use as the pain diminishes.

When I was first becoming aware of the importance of sleep, I treated a fifty-year-old businessman who had experienced chronic neck pain for almost two years. He was the owner of a small accounting firm and was miserable while continuing to work. Extensive physical therapy had not helped. I prescribed a strong sleep medication, which immediately allowed him to sleep a full night. At his two-week follow-up, the medication was working well and the plan was to start him on an aggressive physical therapy program on his next visit. However, eight weeks later, I was surprised to discover that he was pain-free. The power of sleep had never been so apparent and I began to consistently assess my patients' sleep patterns and treat for it.

Although patients will argue with me that it's impossible to sleep with their pain, there are very few situations where the right combination of approaches, including taking sleep medication, won't yield a consistently good night's sleep. These strategies will be discussed in detail in Chapter 11.

## Anxiety

*"It is not true that people stop pursuing dreams because they grow old. They grow old because they stop pursuing dreams."*
Gabriel García Márquez

This is one of my favorite quotes and I see it every day in my practice. However, growing old is not the problem; it is crushing anxiety that destroys your dreams.

Our existence depends on avoiding or minimizing emotional and physical pain and the resultant anxiety. We will go to great lengths to avoid the uncomfortable sensations generated by either one; in doing so, we protect ourselves. Failure elicits feelings of helplessness and vulnerability, and we hate it.

Let's consider our basic needs like air, food, water, shelter and safety. Whenever one of these needs is unmet, we develop an increasing level of anxiety and/ or discomfort, depending on how long it takes to meet the need. Lack of air creates anxiety within seconds, whereas lack of food takes hours. Not being in pain is also a basic human need that is not often discussed.

Humans have the additional capacity to generate anxiety with thoughts. This anxiety is often based on perceived threats; our racing thoughts can disrupt peace of mind indefinitely.

A critical factor in understanding the interaction between mental and physical pain and anxiety is recognizing that it is bi-directional: pain creates anxiety and anxiety increases pain. The interactions happen so fast that it's difficult to really know which came first.

Negative thoughts and physical pain are neurologic links that elicit the physical response and feelings that we describe as anxiety. Because the initial stimulus in this scenario is not anxiety but rather, the mental or physical event, anxiety is not primarily a psychological issue. It is, instead, a programming phenomenon, where both negative thoughts and pain etch in neurological circuits that become stronger with time and repetition, bringing about anxiety each time they are activated. Anxiety then becomes imbedded in the irrational unconscious brain. The unconscious brain processes data many more times per second than the conscious brain. Any time spent solving your anxiety with rational means is a complete mismatch and counter-productive.

### *The Creation of Anxiety*

To further understand anxiety and learn how to handle it effectively, let's look more closely at some of the concepts presented in Chapter 1, The Pathway into Chronic Pain.

Any sensory input can create anxiety. Consider the different types: sight, sound, taste, smell, and touch. Each of them can be perceived as pleasant, neutral, or unpleasant. The unpleasant sensations will create anxiety but they are in the minority; your body processes over 99 percent of them as neutral.[7]

We consciously or unconsciously gravitate toward reward and away from anxiety. For example, a blinding flash of light is a sensory input that will cause you to react and get away from it. If touch is gentle, it can be pleasant, but if increased, it can become painful and at some threshold create anxiety.

Thoughts alone can create anxiety. For example, if you stepped off a curb and almost got hit by a car, your heart might race and your stomach might clench, even though nothing touched you. It was the thought that you might get hit that caused the secretion of chemicals, eliciting the physical response. I think of this sequence as a psychological reflex. In addition to creating anxiety, the reflex sparks a constellation of feelings such as fear, frustration, or anger.

In another example, picture yourself lying on a sunny beach in Hawaii thinking about how glad you are to be on vacation. You feel relaxed because the happy thoughts lead your body to secrete chemicals similar to the drug Valium. Different thoughts can radically change your emotions and physical condition. If you're on the same beach thinking about how poorly your boss has been treating you, how are you going to feel? Probably frustrated and a bit angry. Even though you're on a gorgeous beach, you can't relax. Again, it's the thought, not the circumstances that determines your emotional state. If you continued to think about your bad situation with your boss over and over, it could have the potential to ruin your entire vacation.

This is what happens with chronic pain. Repetitive negative thoughts about your pain produce anxiety and create challenging neurological circuits.

Once the circuits associated with pain are established in your nervous system, they cannot be eliminated. It's possible to influence your own thoughts, however, and create detours around these disconcerting pathways. This is the basis of a branch of psychotherapy called cognitive behavioral therapy (CBT). According to the theory behind CBT you can, through a series of directed exercises, reprogram or re-structure your thinking and improve your mental health. This is a much different process than striving for positive thinking or "mind over matter." There's no way to outrun chronic pain or these relentless circuits.

### *The Natural Progression of Anxiety*

Although anxiety can start with a thought that causes a physiological reaction, there is a step in between. The circuits etched into our minds include images as well as thoughts. A negative thought sparks an image, which then elicits the reflexive anxiety response. The imagery involved can be especially compelling or disruptive, but it occurs so quickly that you may not aware of it.

According to David Burns, author of *Feeling Good*, our anxiety-related thoughts and images are usually based on cognitive distortions—called "errors in thinking"—which then lead to the development of "stories."[8]

A "story" is a preoccupation about some aspect of yourself or circumstance of your life that you think is negative, and often includes self-judgment. "I can't communicate well," "I'm a disorganized person," "I'm bad at relationships"—all examples of common self-judgments. Or it can be about an event that caused you stress: "The doctor did the wrong surgery." Often the story becomes so entrenched that you're convinced it can't be changed.

A friend once had a story about his golf game. He is still a very low handicap golfer in his seventies. He has a beautiful swing that I would love to have a fraction of in my lifetime. He has always been a good golfer; in fact, he played at a national level in his twenties and thirties. These days, he gets frustrated that he's not as good now as he was in his twenties, so he doesn't play as often as he could. When he does, he is quite critical of himself, which detracts from his enjoying his afternoon outside on the course. His "story" of comparing his current game to his prior game is the factor taking away his joy of the game. So far, I have been unsuccessful in getting him to see how he sabotages himself.

Another friend was going through a series of failed relationships a few years ago. Discouraged, he decided that he just wasn't any good at relationships. Every encounter reinforced his story. Instead of working toward developing better skills in this area, he gave up. He became chronically frustrated with everything, which worsened his situation.

The problem with having a "story" is more serious than it would appear on the surface. That's because the story in your head becomes your reality.

An example of a story that morphed into reality occurred one day when I was skiing with one of my son's best friends, Holt, who is essentially part of our family. We were out on a fantastic day in Park City, Utah. My son, Nick, had taken off to practice jumping for his mogul competition. Holt and I were relaxing on the chairlift, but he was not in a great mood. When I asked him what was going on, he told me about an incident that had happened the night before.

A friend of Holt's was being harassed in a bar and when Holt walked over to see what he could do to help, he got physically thrown out by the local police. It was bad enough that the bouncer was acting irrationally, but even worse, the local police had also taken quick action without asking any questions.

As we talked, I pointed out to him that he wasn't really skiing with me; he was so caught up in the story of what had happened that he was still back in the bar. Although his frustrations were justified, he was allowing people he didn't like to take away his ability to enjoy a rare opportunity for us to be able to ski together.

As part of our discussion, we talked about Holt's choices. I had read William Glaser's book, *Choice Theory*[9], a few months earlier. It's an excellent book about how to effectively deal with adverse circumstances. One choice would be to change the circumstances. If you don't have that choice, though, you can change how you relate to them. In Holt's situation, he was bringing the events from the night before to a beautiful ski day. After I pointed this out, he made the choice to either find out the name of the policeman on the case or drop it, and then he could make the choice to enjoy his day.

It was enlightening to watch him go through a little process of acknowledging what was going on and then truly let it go. I could see how the leftover imagery in Holt's head had been his reality at that moment, which gave me a deeper perspective on how this sequence occurs.

Holt did not suppress his frustration. If he had taken that route, those thoughts that had become a story, complete with imagery, would eventually have surfaced and possibly emerged as irrational behavior. It was also interesting to both of us that although we'd talked about these concepts for a couple of years, this situation really brought them home. We ended up having a great time for the rest of the day.

The stories we develop about our lives and ourselves can be deadly to our mental health because we start to interpret random events in a biased way. Many people develop a personal story, casting themselves in a certain role, and then play that role over and over, leaving very little room for wonder and creativity.

With stories about our chronic pain, the stakes are even higher. This is because often the events that started someone on their path to pain are disturbing in themselves. Once this is added to an unpleasant physical sensation—which intensifies the repetition of every detail—it's not unlikely that the rest of our bad luck in life will get blamed on those circumstances, whether they're related or not. Multiple research papers demonstrate that many people in chronic pain are still upset with the person, employer, or situation that had caused their injury. One of the problems with "external attribution" is that we feel even more helpless and experience even more pain.[10]

One of my chronic pain patients, a fifty-year-old man, had been hit head-on by a drunk driver of a semi-truck. My patient's major injuries, including a pelvic fracture, had healed; but he was still suffering from severe low back pain. Although the accident had occurred five years earlier, he talked about it like it had happened yesterday. It had become the central story of his life. He had given up control of his existence to the negligent truck driver.

What are your stories? What imagery do you have in your mind about yourself, your family, spouse, work, and so on?

### *Societal Reinforcement of Anxiety*

We've established that thoughts awaken or produce images that cause the body to respond reflexively. Much, if not most, of human behavior is centered on minimizing the unpleasant feelings associated with anxiety. Therefore, others can manipulate you by creating or reinforcing anxiety-provoking situations. Consider how anxiety-inducing imagery is used to influence our behavior.

### Marketing

The marketing world has a major impact on our anxiety. A marketer's goal is to produce images of what we should own, look like, or experience in order to be happy and fulfilled. The subtler (or not-so-subtle) message is that we are inadequate human beings if we don't own the things they want us to buy. In other words, if we feel bad enough about ourselves, we'll take action in the form of purchasing goods or experiences to decrease our anxiety. These days, we are constantly exposed to intense marketing imagery. It's impossible to escape it without becoming a recluse.

I realized a few years ago that every human being has some level of a body image disorder. You might be fine or like 99 percent of your physical appearance but it's unlikely that you will love every millimeter of it. What happens is that if you think about it, you are now reinforcing the negative circuits. If you suppress these thoughts, they become much stronger. Since you cannot escape your body, the repetition becomes endless and progressive over time. As you are trapped, you may become increasingly frustrated, which really fires up your nervous system and adrenaline/cortisol levels. It is all a neurological trick; and tools to work on self-acceptance will have little impact on this process. You can resort to cosmetic surgery but invariably your brain will find another body part to focus on.

Then the marketing world piles on to this problem by making you feel even worse. The imagery presented to us in the media is unattainable for most of us. Now, with digital touching up of photos, even the models themselves cannot attain what's being presented as ideal to the masses. We also rarely see the models without their makeup or styling; in reality, they don't look so much different from the rest of us mortals. It's fascinating to me to see how the professional makeup artists can make almost anyone look remarkably good.

The magnification of body image problems has many negative effects on society. Eating disorders have reached epidemic proportions. In a 2004 Norwegian study, almost one in five females had experienced an eating disorder, and this is also becoming a male issue.[11] Men have historically taken a different tack in the form of aggressive bodybuilding. I remember in seventh grade being ecstatic when my parents bought me a set of weights so I could transform my scarecrow frame. (Didn't work.) These days, obesity is at an epidemic level for both genders. There are many causes, but I think one factor is that people feel anxious about not having the body they want and about the difficulty of achieving their ideal. The emotional energy needed to go and exercise, organize a diet, and more, gets burned up in a cycle of anxiety and frustration.

Consider the market created by not feeling good about one's body: the industries based on solving the problem with diets, exercise programs, makeup, clothes, or plastic surgery. The list seems endless. If the anxiety could be more successfully tolerated, the need for these products and services would rapidly diminish.

The resultant problem is twofold. The media imagery becomes more intense over time, both with marketing techniques and in our minds; and we become less equipped to resist. It becomes increasingly difficult to remain unphased by these crushing irrational circuits.

### Familial Imprinting

During the first ten to twelve years of your life, your immediate environment is downloaded into your brain. That database will go on to have a profound effect on your adult life and sense of well-being. Although many mental health problems have a genetic basis, the early programming of the brain is a significant factor.

In 1960, a man named Robert Hoffman developed the concept he termed *negative love syndrome.* In the negative love syndrome, a child instinctively adopts most if not all of his parents' behavioral patterns in order to be accepted and loved. It's both an emotional and physical survival tool. Hoffman started a program that evolved into the Hoffman Process, in which participants learn how to become aware of these patterns. The first step is to identify the dysfunctional patterns of each parent; next, you identify your own. Before doing the Hoffman Process, I'd spent many years working on myself and was shocked to discover these patterns were controlling my actions.

This seven-day in-house program is designed to give you the tools to recognize and process these patterns so they no longer run your life. It allowed me to connect to my own personal value system and to separate myself from my background on a certain level. This is an example of reprogramming that we discussed earlier in the chapter.

Anxiety in its many forms is a predominant pattern that's passed on to us from our families of origin. Our parents do imprint positive, loving patterns upon us, but unfortunately, as life progresses, there is more reinforcement of the negative patterns. Life generally does not get easier as we move through it.

Any time you feel anxiety you are in a preprogrammed pattern. The Hoffman tools allow you to choose your response to any given situation instead of having a predictable, unmediated response. The Hoffman Process also dramatically organized my thinking in a way that allowed me to write this book.

### Cultural Programming

Throughout world history, rulers have used fear to control populations. The bully we all feared and hated in school is often in charge. Released from the constraints of adolescence, these rulers typically come to power using the same techniques they employed on the playground.

A big difference between schoolyard days and adulthood is that the people in charge use visually brutal tactics to subjugate the population. There are endless examples throughout history and still ongoing: Rulers throughout history have used systematic torture and death squads to subjugate conquered or rebellious territories. Millions of women underwent the Catholic Church's trial by torture to determine if they were witches during the Dark Ages. Gangs keep their "soldiers" in line with torture. In this day and age of the internet we are all even more connected to atrocities by imagery. Much, if not most, of the world's population is still controlled by fear.

Fear factors deeply into our programming. It's reinforced by traumatic events such as the Great Depression, the two World Wars, and 9/11. The impact of these events can last a lifetime. My parents' behavior was permanently affected by the Depression era. Most of my friends from Holocaust families feel that it is almost impossible for their parents and grandparents to thrive.

### The Myth of Self-Esteem

Self-esteem is one of the worst concepts ever propagated in the human experience. It implies that if you have enough of "X"—a great job, beautiful house, physically attractive partner, for example—then you'll think well of yourself and have less anxiety, less frustration, and more happiness.

Self-esteem is a subtle form of masking. Scoring achievements and gaining possessions doesn't help you get rid of anxiety or anger; they only cover them up. It's trying to get rid of anxiety through rational means; you think that once you have everything you thought you always wanted, there will be no more reason to feel anxious or mad. But there's one big problem with this: you can't successfully deal with these powerful irrational pathways of anxiety with rational thinking. There's a huge mismatch.

Self-esteem actually worsens your anxiety levels: when you've reached the pinnacle of our society's version of success but you're still suffering from anxiety, then where do you go? What do you do next? Now you are really lost.

Our society has taken the cult of self-esteem even further. We're so focused on winning that many of us cease to really enjoy the experience or the activity at hand. Winning is fine. But remember only a small percent of individuals can win in any given scenario.

I've seen the downside of focusing on winning via my son Nick and his friend Holt, who are world-class mogul skiers. During training, both were so (understandably) set on clinching first place that it compromised their day-to-day enjoyment of the activity itself. I often spoke to both of them about how winning an Olympic medal or a national championship wouldn't have much impact on their lives in the long run; it was more important to appreciate and enjoy the whole act of competing.

In 2007, Holt won the national championship in mogul skiing, an achievement he readily attributes, at least in part, to the awareness and visualization techniques presented in this book. Much of his success, he said, was due to letting go of the outcome and performing with freedom. The more focused he was on winning, the less consistent his performance was. The day after his victory, he turned to me and to his performance coach, David Elaimy, and said, "You were right. Winning changed my life for about twelve hours. Life moves on."

*It's excellent to strive for excellence and be a productive human being, but it has nothing to do with decreasing your anxiety and frustrations.*

Self-esteem involves self-judgment. Whether it's positive or negative, judgment, directed at yourself or others, prevents you from being fully aware of what's immediately in front of you.

### The Lifetime Progression of Anxiety

Untreated anxiety will always progress. I can't make that point strongly enough. The natural progression of anxiety is:

- Alertness (normal, appropriate response to a situation)
- Nervousness
- General anxiety (being a worrier)
- Anxiety reactions
    - Exaggerated physical responses
    - Panic attacks
- Obsessive Compulsive Disorder (OCD)

### Coping with Anxiety

Some of the coping mechanisms we use are:

- Suppression and denial
- Rigid, structured thinking
- Avoiding anxiety-producing situations
    - Phobias
    - Decreasing the "size" of one's life

- Masking
  - Addictions
  - Distractions
- Pursuit of power
  - Gaining strength
    - Physical
    - Mental
    - Spiritual
    - Financial
- Controlling
  - People
    - Marriage
    - Children and household
  - Employer/employee

What percent of successful people are driven by anxiety, and mask it, instead of being driven by a vision based on love?

Many of the above endeavors are worthwhile and greatly contribute to one's quality of life and the welfare of society. However, if the drive to pursue them is anxiety-based instead of love-based, then the consequences can be significant.

Mind you, many of us have coping methods that do not interrupt our lives. For instance, a businesswoman friend once asked me to dinner specifically to discuss her own tactics in light of the stress management concepts that I teach. She was curious because while she was not experiencing much anxiety, she did have certain habits, like brushing her teeth a specific way and doing counting rituals. She was aware that her behavior was a little odd. After talking to her for a while, I realized that she was living a pretty reasonable life. The business she owned was quite successful but purposefully kept small. Her strategies for keeping anxiety at bay were working. From my point of view, it didn't look like she needed to make any significant changes or embark on new endeavors.

Many coping strategies are effective. However, I assume that if you are reading this book, then the elephant still in the room is that you are experiencing mental or physical pain and your life is not as fulfilling and happy as you would like.

I frequently encounter patients who are in crippling, severe pain, are completely disabled, and yet rank themselves as a zero on the anxiety, depression, and irritability scales on my spine intake questionnaire. Their anxiety-suppressing mechanisms have worked: they are disconnected from their own anxiety. But you can't be disconnected from your anxiety and be connected to yourself. I am rarely able to break through this wall, and very few of them engage in the DOC (Define your Own Care) process. Even if you had a perfect life and were not affected by societal pressures, just being in chronic pain provides enough stress. Now that we understand the link between emotional and physical pain, it is clear that pain will be expressed in some manner. Almost every person has at least three to five of the NPD symptoms listed in Chapter 1.

### *Am I Operating on Your Pain or Your Anxiety?*

My decision-making process in terms of whether to recommend surgery or not has become clearer over the last couple of years—but in an unexpected way. It turns out that diminishing anxiety is a bigger concern than alleviating pain. I had no idea.

Surgeons are trained to focus on addressing pain. Although they are aware of other factors that can adversely affect outcomes, they tend to ignore them. It has been documented that less than 10 percent of surgeons assess stress before making a final decision regarding surgery.[12] We also do not take sleep into account, which has, as discussed, has a profound impact on pain.[13]

A series of cases brought to light how often patients think that surgery will get rid of their anxiety. Not long ago, I had an almost identical conversation with four patients, each of whom had leg pain. I thought the structural problems were severe enough that we commenced discussing surgical options. All were men between the ages of forty-five and sixty-five with leg pain originating from an identifiable problem in their spines. The pain was severe enough that each also wanted to undergo surgery. However, they all measured at least an eight out of ten on the anxiety scale and were not sleeping well. Their stresses included seriously ill family members, loss of jobs, marital problems, etc., and understandably, none of them were coping that well.

Each patient was familiar with the DOC program but had not mean-ingfully engaged with the concepts. They were coming back for their second and third visits. Finally, I asked each of them the same question: "What would it be like if I could surgically solve the pain in your leg but the anxiety you are experiencing would continue to progress over the next thirty to forty years?" Their eyes widened with a panicked look and each one replied, "That would not be OK. I could not live like this." Each of them also grabbed his leg and asked, "Won't getting rid of this pain alleviate my anxiety?"

My answer was no. Anxiety is a core symptom of the neurophysiologic disorder and the circuits associated with it are permanent. Chronic pain is a huge stressor that reinforces those neurological pathways. Although relieving the stress of pain will usually temporarily decrease anxiety, it will remain a significant long-term problem. There are too many other life situations that fuel anxiety.

I told each patient that although I would love to use surgery to get rid of their leg pain, my bigger concern was their severe anxiety and possibly chronic pain. I recalled my fifteen-year battle with pain and anxiety during which I was on an endless quest to find the *one* single answer that would solve everything—both my pain and anxiety. I also remembered the intensity of that need. Raw anxiety is intolerable.

Then I asked each of them, "If I could resolve your anxiety but you would have to live with your leg pain, what would that be like?" Although not completely happy about the scenario, they thought they could deal with it. It was more palatable than experiencing no abatement of their fear.

Once I gained this awareness of the crippling effects of anxiety I began to systematically implement a pre-operative process that I call "prehab." Why prehab? Because, for decades, the medical literature has shown that there are clear risk factors to having poor surgical results. They include lack of sleep, high-dose narcotic use, anxiety, anger, catastrophizing, fear-avoidance, depression, loss of job, family stress, poor physical conditioning, and pre-existing chronic pain in any other part of the body. Prehab consists of having patients engage in the DOC process for eight to twelve weeks prior to elective surgery.

The progress does not have to be perfect. I just want my patients to possess a basic understanding of pain before undergoing a procedure, as well as begin to address these known factors that compromise outcomes.

The barometer I use before I help them make the final surgical decision is whether they are sleeping well, their anxiety levels have dropped, and they are actively engaged in expressive writing, which I will discuss later. My experience with performing surgery on a patient with a fired-up nervous system has consistently been less than satisfactory. Pain control is difficult and even the longer-term results are marginal, as there is often a significant amount of residual pain.

What happened after I started incorporating the DOC process was completely unexpected. Many of my patients with severe structural problems would come in for their final pre-operative visit and cancel surgery because the pain had disappeared.

## Back to Hunting Elk

Herbert, in his mid-sixties, had been experiencing severe leg pain for over a year. His pain had progressed to the level where he had to get around in a wheelchair, and he was not very happy, especially in light of how active he was. His MRI showed a severe constriction of his spine between his third and fourth lumbar vertebrae and also his fourth and fifth level. Normally, a spinal canal is 15mm in diameter and symptoms often occur when the canal narrows down to 8 or 9mm. It is similar to the narrow part of an hourglass. His canal was down to 4mm and I was concerned enough that I rearranged my schedule in order to do surgery earlier. He also was not buying this chronic pain explanation and would not engage in the expressive writing. He came down with a respiratory infection and we had to delay his surgery.

When I called him about the need to delay his operation, I said, "Herbert, humor me. At least start with the expressive writing and look at my book." He grudgingly agreed. I got a phone call about a week later that he was feeling better. I asked him if he still wanted to have the surgery. He said he did. There was no question in my mind that it needed to be done. The Friday before his Monday surgery he cancelled it because his pain was gone. I talked to him about three months later and he was back in the hills hunting elk. Several years later he is still doing fine. Every patient who has cancelled surgery has had severe pathology. I've never performed surgery on patients with mild or moderate problems. It has become unclear to me who I should be operating on, so I just plan on getting the best outcomes with or without surgery.

## The Modifiers—Sleep and Anxiety—Final Thoughts

Chronic pain and how to deal with it in their patients frustrates most physicians because they feel it is unsolvable. When I lecture to audiences of physicians, I ask, "How many enjoy treating patients suffering from chronic pain?" Very few raise their hands. I recently addressed a group of over a hundred primary care physicians and not one raised their hand. The same holds true for anxiety-related disorders. Although there have been many advances in managing the symptoms of anxiety, severe anxiety-related disorders such as bipolar disorder and obsessive-compulsive disorder (OCD) have poor prognoses in terms of a cure. These disorders are symptoms of permanent, powerful irrational neurological pathways. It doesn't work to attempt to "fix" them with a psychological model.

One research paper documented that alternative medicine is more effective than traditional Western medicine in treating chronic pain.[14] This is not surprising, as these approaches tend to revolve around calming down the nervous system, which would decrease the body's stress response.

Mental and physical pain both stimulate the secretion of stress hormones, which create anxiety. These chemicals change the pain threshold, which increases the intensity of the pain. Sleep changes both the perception of pain and your capacity to cope with it. Anger is an additional modifier that will be discussed in the next chapter.

# CHAPTER 5

---

# The Ultimate Modifier—Anger

*Our afflictions are not imposed by the Divine.*
*Rather, they lead us to the Divine more often than our joys do.*
*Do not resist the bitter pills in your life;*
*know that they will lead you to a greater awareness.*
—Bernie Siegel

MOST OF MY PATIENTS ARE UPSET AND ANGRY ABOUT SUFFERING from unending pain, and who can blame them? Chronic pain drastically alters every aspect of your life in a terrible way. It would be enough to make anyone angry. But if you'd like to eliminate your pain and be able to flourish, it's vital you address your anger. If you ignore it, it will entrap you and take you to an even worse place, caught in a vicious circle: your pain makes you angry and your anger worsens your pain. In this chapter, we will look at how anger develops and how it influences chronic pain.

We have discussed how, when a basic human need such as eating, drinking, or breathing isn't met, we experience anxiety, which triggers action to resolve the problem. If our attempts fail, our body kicks in with adrenaline, which increases the odds of us meeting our needs. The net result is anger, which occurs because of our loss of control. (Anger is anxiety with a chemical kick.) With anger your body is now fully adrenalized.

To be able to live pain-free is a basic human need. The vast majority of the time, pain triggers a rapid protective response and the pain disappears. With chronic pain, however, the pain never disappears; you are trapped in a constant fight-or-flight mode. Additionally, there does not seem to be a way out, and life turns dark—very dark. My patients cannot find words to describe the depth of their suffering and despair.

## The Genealogy of Anger

There is a sequence of events that causes anger:

1. Circumstance (real or imagined)
2. Blame
3. Victimhood
4. Frustration and anger

In this sequence, you blame a person or circumstance for disrupting your sense of well-being, which places you in the role of a victim, and you become angry.

The blame-victim-anger sequence can start with either a perceived wrong or an actual wrong. When it's a perceived wrong, it's easy to be misled by your thought process. Your mind creates a story about the event, but there's a good chance that the triggering event wasn't a "real" wrong. Examples include being cut off in traffic or being inadvertently left off a party list. Even if it was a random act, you feel victimized. Whatever thoughts or imagery exist in your mind will create your version of reality and you become upset.

In the second scenario, you have genuinely been wronged. You might have been robbed or assaulted. Your surgery went horribly wrong and then you found out that it probably should have never been performed. A driver ran a red light and totaled your car. Here, you are a victim in the truest sense.

Whether the victim role is perceived or actual, the anger response will be the same. The imagery in your mind from the perceived wrong will elicit as strong a response as being treated badly, so both scenarios are equally destructive to your health and sense of well-being. The difference is that when you actually are a victim, it's much harder to let go of that role. This puts you at a disadvantage, because you cannot experience the full benefit of forgiveness until you forgive the person who has wronged you the most.

Playing the victim is a universal part of the human experience, since none of us has complete freedom of action. We are limited by:

- Basic survival needs
- Money
- Time
- Physical attributes and conditions (appearance, intelligence, abilities)
- Opportunity

How you relate to your limitations, including chronic pain, determines whether or not you place yourself in the victim role.

There are some people who resist playing the victim even under extreme circumstances. Consider the life of Nelson Mandela. Unjustly imprisoned for twenty-five years, he forgave his captors and went on to become a gracious statesman. He even put some of his former captors to work in his security force.

An almost incomprehensible story is that of Viktor Frankl, a Jewish Austrian psychiatrist and author of *Man's Search for Meaning.*[1] Frankl, who survived three years in World War II concentration camps, was at one point slated to undergo human medical experimentation. Instead of going into the victim role, he asked himself the question, "What is life asking of me right now?"

I once had a patient who suffered a terrible complication after a major spine operation, one that resulted in permanent blindness. Somehow the blood supply to the optic nerve had been compromised during the procedure. Everyone was shocked, as the surgery had initially seemed to go so well. About three months later he walked into my office and said to me, "This is the hand I've been dealt. I'm going to play it." I saw him again eight years later to remove his spinal implants. He was still completely blind, had gone through a bitter divorce, and had experienced several significant financial setbacks. However, he still had the same proactive mindset.

## The Abyss

There are many phases in the evolution of chronic pain and it is not a linear journey. When circumstances are easier, then life is simply better. Situational stresses can pull you down for days or weeks, and then you can rebound. However, chronic unrelenting pain will pull you down and over time, patients in chronic pain usually hit a tipping point where they fall into a dark mental state that I call "the Abyss."

In the Abyss, you have lost control of almost everything, including pain, finances, full participation in physical activities, and enjoying leisure pursuits. Other aspects living in the Abyss include:

- Friends, family, peers, employers, and health care providers often do not believe you are suffering that much. The disbelief seems to worsen as you try to convince them.

- You might be at the mercy of a claims manager who has little medical training and no concept of how your life is being affected by your pain.
- You may have undergone a failed operation or series of operations. You are angry about the outcome and the events that led you to decide to have the surgery in the first place, but you cannot go back.

Multiply all of this by time, and I think you will get the picture. Not only is there repetition of anxiety, pain, and frustration, there is also usually no known endpoint and no hope of escape.

Viktor Frankl described his incomprehensible ordeal in detail. He pointed out that the worst part of it was not the hardship itself, but not knowing if and when there would be an end. Sound familiar?

Suffering from unrelenting pain is like having your soul pounded into the ground by a pile driver. Your life is being systematically destroyed. You may have achieved a full and successful life only to have it consumed by pain. The dark place that develops in and envelops your mind is deep. My patients cannot find words to describe the depth of frustration they feel being in the Abyss. I was in this hole for fifteen years and I will never forget any aspect of it.

## Falling into the Abyss

It is anger that ushers you into the Abyss and anger that keeps you there. People intellectually know that being chronically angry, as most chronic pain patients understandably are, is not a great way to live life. Yet a high percentage of the population lives in this state. There are over 100 million people in the U.S. alone suffering from chronic pain.[2] There are many ways to fall into and remain in the Abyss, including:

- Needing validation
- Disguising your anger from others and yourself
- Choosing to remain a victim
- Failing to recognize that the Abyss is your baseline state
- Being a perfectionist
- Losing hope

### *Needing Validation*

The need to be validated causes and drives frustration. It is much stronger than you can perceive. Our need to be validated begins as soon as we have consciousness and a sense of self. Without an identifiable source of pain on a test, patients feel that no one believes their pain is real. I do understand my patients are in pain, whether or not I can find a cause. However, they become understandably obsessive about the possibility that something serious has been missed because their suffering is so extreme.

Surgeons generally think mechanically and conversations with them inevitably focus on identifying the cause. When one isn't found, the surgeon also may not believe that the pain is real. Anybody will get fired up over not being believed, and now the actual pain becomes worse because the individual is flooded with stress chemicals. The mission to find an answer will escalate. The term I used for myself in this phase was "epiphany addict." I was convinced that I just needed to find the one answer to my problems.

At some point in the pursuit of validation rational thinking simply disappears. Sadly, patients' all-consuming preoccupation to find the answer shuts out others—even those close to them. They shut down and are no longer open to new ideas. This is the major block to healing.

A surgical scar can be validating, no matter the outcome of the surgery. In Dr. Peter Fritzell's study looking at patients who had undergone fusion for low back pain versus nonoperative care, 16 percent of the patients who did poorly stated that they would choose to undergo the surgery again.[3] A scar on one's back is a strong justification for suffering.

### Disguising Your Anger

No one likes the idea of being a victim, so we suppress or disconnect from taking on that role. There are many creative ways to be a victim and also endless ways to conceal it, both from others and from one's self. Here are some of the ways:

- Having strong opinions—being "right"
- Feeling sorry for yourself
- Suppressing negative thoughts
- Dissociating—closing the door on the past—experiencing a "new beginning"
- Identifying yourself as "cool and calm"
- Being perfectionistic and judgmental

As you become more honest with yourself and recognize your victimhood, you can at least give yourself a little credit for creativity. I joke with my patients that disguising my anger is my most highly developed life skill.

One of many examples of "feeling sorry for myself" occurred one afternoon I spent with my wife while visiting Yosemite. My wife and I were leaving the park. I will preface this story by letting you know that my wife is a true city girl. She is the only person I know who would go hiking with me in high-heeled sneakers and a mini-skirt. Although she lived in the Bay Area, only about four hours' drive away, she'd never been to Yosemite. She was very concerned about the bears and all of the bear warning signs did not help to allay her anxiety. I had been going there for years and earnestly assured her that bears weren't very active during the day and weren't going to be a problem.

The first day, as we were just beginning a hike, we met a couple of women at the Vernal Fall Bridge. One of them was an avid nature photographer and excitedly told us how she had seen three bears in the last two days. At that moment I lost all credibility with my wife.

Two days later, we were leaving the Ahwahnee Hotel on the floor of the valley on what couldn't have been a clearer or more beautiful day. The road to Glacier Point had just opened and there were very few people out. As we got into the car, my wife made a comment about the bear warning sign in front of the hotel. From her perspective, her comment was a light joke. But I took it personally as an assault on my character. Instead of letting it go, I held on to it and stopped talking to her. I was feeling very sorry for myself. The ensuing conversation was one I wouldn't have chosen for such a wonderful drive. I couldn't let go of the fact that "she was the one who started it all" and blamed her for ruining our drive.

Fortunately, when it comes to these types of conflicts, my wife is a little wiser than I am. She wasn't thrilled with me, but talked to me in a way that helped me see that I was playing the victim. I'm thankful for the people in my life, like my wife, who can give me a reality check.

I'd like to say that I was never again the source of that kind of tension between my wife and me; however, that's not the case. I do consider these situations to be learning experiences, though, and try to use them to avoid similar exchanges in the future. Doing so will only affect my relationships and quality of life in a positive way.

Another recurring example of my tendency to fall into victimhood was when I repeatedly told my wife that I needed to write this book but was working too hard and didn't have enough time. I felt justified in these feelings until I finally realized that I was allowing myself to be a victim of circumstances and the clock. I had three choices. One was to continue to complain and remain agitated. Another was to forget about the book, taking it off of my to-do list. A third was to write and finish the book. That insight allowed me to realize how much of my energy was being drained by not taking full responsibility for my actions.

### "I Am Not Angry"

My patients rate themselves on my intake questionnaire on a zero-to-ten scale with regards to anxiety, depression, and irritability (anger). I frequently observe them rank themselves as a zero on all three variables. In these cases, I am rarely successful in helping them resolve their pain. I will still give it my best shot but there is nothing I can say that will motivate them to engage in the DOC process. The elephant in the room, of course, is that they are experiencing chronic pain.

An article by Allan Abbass[4] succinctly points out that if you are disconnected from this set of negative emotions, then you will experience symptoms in other parts of your body. Everyone has anxiety; it is necessary for survival. But you cannot solve a problem that you are not aware of having.

A few months ago, I evaluated a retired attorney for pain down the front of his right leg. It had begun about eight months earlier. The pain was moderate but frustrating. He had not experienced prior back problems and was not used to dealing with pain. It was unclear what might have precipitated this pain. His wife, a retired businesswoman, accompanied him.

My intake form consists of twelve pages. It includes questions about sleep, stress, work, as well as medical and family issues. He had only filled out the part of the form dealing with his spine pain and medical problems, skipping any questions that dealt with personal issues. The MRI of his lower back revealed some small bone spurs, but they were on the opposite side of his body than his pain. I did not have a structural explanation for his symptoms.

I explained that I needed to have him fill out the rest of the intake questionnaire before I could fully engage in the interview. I returned five minutes later and he stated that he did not want to fill the personal profile section because he was not a chronic pain patient.

It took me about ten minutes to explain that even if there was a structural problem, I felt that surgery was only part of the solution. Rehab, conditioning, and dealing with the central nervous system was important for a good outcome with or without surgery. I wished to give him the best chance at a good result. I hadn't addressed the fact that I did not see a surgical lesion and I needed to order more tests.

He started to scream at me that he was not angry and that all he needed was an operation to solve the problem and to get on with his life. He had a long vacation planned in three weeks. He turned to his wife and said, "Well, what do you think about what he is saying?" Her reply was, "I think you had better listen to him." I finally had to bring in my most experienced nurse to talk to him. She could not calm him down and I offered to have him see one of my partners.

### *Remaining a Victim*
Being a victim is one of the deepest rooted human behavioral patterns, one that is dramatically reinforced in the presence of chronic pain. Here are the "benefits" of playing the victim:

- Others expect less of you
- You expect less of yourself
- You feel powerful, which masks feeling vulnerable
- It gives you a sense of entitlement
- You "justifiably" manipulate those around you
- You possess a sense of conviction and being "right"

Being treated poorly by the Workers' Compensation system is victimhood in the truest sense. You have little, if any, say in the way the claim is being run and you have lost control of your entire life. The only control you often have is to remain in the victim role. If you are angry with your employer, you can really stick it to them with the cost of your medical care. Why get better? No one really seems to care. However, choosing victimhood instead of getting better doesn't work. Your employer will survive. Your claims examiner will go to work tomorrow. There's not one person you're going to permanently harm. Yet you have allowed chronic anger to erode your quality of life.

I know that it's hard to commit to a different way of living. We all have familiar patterns, and it makes us anxious to give them up. There's comfort in being a victim. Somehow we are willing to continue to suffer rather than change—the anxiety associated with change may feel worse than remaining in your current circumstances. There have been numerous studies done on chronic illness, which show that patients drop out of treatment 30 to 50 percent of the time. It does not seem to depend on the success of the treatment.[5]

Choosing to remain a victim is the biggest obstacle to healing, since it is such a powerful role. Most people never want to give it up. In order to go through the DOC process, however, you have to make a simple intellectual choice to give it up and often make this choice multiple times a day.

Anger is one of the symptoms of NPD that blocks treatment. Your brain is spinning so fast that you have difficulty seeing alternatives and become fixated on finding a cause for your pain and getting it fixed.

### Failing to Recognize that Victim is your Baseline

I was unaware that I have lived most of my life playing the victim until age fifty, as my baseline reality was being raised in an abusive household. Only through extensive counseling did I realize that my childhood was not the norm. Each mental health professional I encountered pointed out that the abuse I endured was severe.

What is now disturbing to me is that I would frequently tell others that my parents really loved us. I do know that my mother deeply cared for us but she had no control over her rage. After its two- or three-day course had run, she was incredibly apologetic and complimentary. However, her words would not nearly make up for the mental and physical damage that she had inflicted on us. In my mind, violence and love were mixed together and it was confusing.

Another case of love mixing with violence was a situation that my friend, Sheila, witnessed at the grocery store. Sheila was standing in the checkout line when she heard a young mother screaming at her five-year-old daughter to put something back on the shelf. She suddenly hauled off and slapped her child with a full swing. Almost instantly, the young girl began to cry, held out her arms, and ran to her mother for comfort. Who else was there to console her? Talk about becoming crosswired—the girl's source of pain was also her bastion of love and protection.

I did not have any close friends until I was in seventh grade. I never hung out with other friends and their families. It was only when I was exposed to more functional families that I began to understand the severity of my mother's pathology.

I thought my chaotic family story was unusual until I attended an event at the Hyde School, where my daughter went for her junior and senior years of high school. Located in Bath, Maine, the school is unique in that the founder, Joey Gauld, made character development the highest priority. It also offers an excellent academic program, in addition to the arts and athletics. The students meet regularly and challenge one another to reach for their highest individual potential. The families participate in group meetings three times during the year.

At my first Joey Gauld seminar in 2007, I was in a large circle with about fifteen other parents. Gauld asked the question, "What problems do you think your family passed on to you that you may have passed on to your child?" and gave each of us five minutes to answer. He was eighty years old at the time and an amazing individual. In five to ten minutes he would assess the issue and give priceless pearls of insight.

As we went around the circle, I was shocked to hear that all but one parent had endured various forms of abusive upbringing, including neglect, alcoholic rages, emotional and physical abuse, and more. It was interesting to note that every parent in the circle had a successful career. Whether they were CEOs of huge corporations or working in a smaller arena, it did not matter. The stories were dismal. Only then did I realize that sharing my personal struggles under the guise of "helping" others was yet another way of remaining in the victim role. Five years after I thought I had given up the victim role, I was still deeply in it.

### *Being a Perfectionist: A Common Victim Role*

Many view perfection as the standard that must be reached in order to be successful. It's held up as a virtue in all aspects of our lives, especially in professional and vocational endeavors. We feel pressure from others to be perfect, and we pressure ourselves.

Perfection does not exist in the human experience. The closest thing to perfection I see is in the nature and design of the human body. A newborn baby is beyond wonder.

Perfection fits into the anger cascade in the following manner. A given situation, person, or yourself, are less than your concept of ideal. You blame one of the above for being "less than perfect." You are now a victim of "less than perfect" and perpetually in some state of conscious or unconscious agitation. Dr. David Burns in his book, *Ten Days to Self-Esteem,* points out that the gap between your concept of perfect and your reality is the degree of your unhappiness.[6]

Since perfection is unattainable, why do so many of us continue to embrace it?[7] I will offer a couple of observations from the perspective of an extreme perfectionist. First of all, we are programmed to be all that we can be. We are also taught that pushing yourself is the best way to accomplish this goal—except that pushing evolves into punishing in the form of self-criticism. Since this strategy often achieves impressive short- and medium-term results, it seems like a reasonable pathway. It's not. The same driving energy that pushes you up the hill takes you down the other side.

I feel a second factor is that the victim role is so powerful that many people find it hard to part with.

It appears that one of the unspoken goals people have is to attain a permanent pain-free state. They do not realize that mental and physical pain are one and the same. A stress-free life isn't possible. Many patients return to my office almost euphoric that they are free of pain. The first words out of my mouth are, "Prepare to fail." These pain pathways are permanent and you will continually hit triggers that will set them off. Your pain will return at the same or worse intensity as before. If you are still holding onto *perfect*, you will be further disappointed and upset. The DOC project is about letting go, allowing yourself to fail, and moving on. Perfect does not allow for failure.

## Perfectionism Seems to Be Everywhere

A friend of mine recently lost his wife. He's a high-level professional and is trying to meet someone to start a new life. Invariably he becomes upset over feeling inadequate, not being a good conversationalist, having interests that are too narrow, not liking his appearance... the list goes on. Then it came out that he places these same labels on his dates. What he is not aware of, is that our minds project onto other people and situations the way we feel about ourselves. This is psychology 101.

The term is "projection." So when you are in a judgmental mode and expressing it to others, you are revealing to the world the way you feel about yourself. This is particularly true if you are upset.

Anthony de Mello, in his book *The Way to Love*[8], points out that eventually you learn to thank the person who upset you because they are the window into your own soul. If you are hard on yourself, you will be critical of others and you cannot unlink these circuits. The other person simply triggered you and they are not what is upsetting you. This concept is the most difficult part of this whole journey for me because it still feels like it is them and not me. This is especially true with spouses.

Another friend is extremely self-critical. He cannot accept any part of himself or enjoy the results of his excellent work. He is still suffering from chronic low back pain and searching the planet for an answer. His lower back MRI is normal for his age. His endless quest is time-consuming and expensive. Meanwhile, he stopped his expressive writing, was only doing a little meditation, and was not sleeping well. He had discontinued the basics that he had experienced some success with. When you stop using the strategies that you know are helpful, it's self-destructive.

When I asked him the same question about being hard on himself, he could barely put into words how critical he is with both himself and those close to him. He could not forgive himself for some of his past behaviors. Then I asked him, "What do you really want? Do you want to be pain free? Or would you rather remain in this self-vindictive angry state of mind and continue to suffer in pain?" It caught him off guard. He was making his own life miserable as well as his family members'.

Whether you verbalize it or not, people know when they are being judged. I challenged him to give up the victim role or move on and at least not subject his family to his self-directed anger. I don't know the end of this story yet.

The fallout of this endless self-criticism, and therefore criticism of others, is devastating to families and also to our society. I am talking to many of my friends' children who have ideals for themselves that cannot be met. It's perverse in an era of so much opportunity that our children feel so pressured to be all that they can be. Why not teach them to enjoy themselves and let who they are simply evolve?

Chronic pain is now an epidemic amongst teenagers. I lectured at a local high school and learned that over 20 percent of the students were on some type of medication for a chronic illness. What's going on?

I had one conversation with a 25-year-old girl who had developed a severe case of OCD. Her anxiety had begun in middle school and manifested itself by overdoing homework to the point where she could not complete it. Her OCD had become progressively worse and now she could not hold a job. Yet she was personable, attractive, and competent.

What happened is that her story of not being good enough or perfect became its own reality. It was a circuit that had become deeply etched into her brain, similar to phantom limb pain. I call it "phantom brain pain." It is not rational, and strategies such as increasing your self-esteem or overachieving will not turn off this noise. I shared my story about how deeply I was in this hole and am now thriving. The conversation seemed helpful to her and she is beginning to heal.

So what is the solution? I would like to present one principle regarding solving perfectionism—*get happy*. One of my remarkably successful mentors reminded me of an important principle regarding success and achievement. First commit to being happy, as it is a learned skill. Then, create a vision of where you want to go.

Creating a vision of excellence is much different than having "high standards." You understand and accept where you are along with your resources. Then you create a plan to get there. Part of this involves filling your brain with positive solutions as well as accepting the inevitable failures. This is a different journey from wasting your energy flagellating yourself for your inadequacies and failures. If you are not willing to fail, then don't attempt the journey. Paradoxically, you will have an endless amount of additional energy to achieve your goals. Happiness is only possible while pursuing a vision of excellence.

### Losing Hope

Harry Harlow was an internationally renowned psychologist who pioneered research in human maternal-infant bonding using primates. Dr. Harlow was the leading force in developing the attachment theory using various species of monkeys.[9]

He turned his attention, also based on primate research, to some of the smaller details of human interaction. One model he worked on was inducing depression. He used various isolation methods and ways of simulating parental neglect or even abuse. He was able to consistently produce monkeys that were seriously disturbed, but he was not able to cause depression.

He finally discovered a methodology where he devised an apparatus that resembled an upside-down pyramid, with a mesh cover. The sides were steep but still allowed the monkey to climb to the top to peek outside. For the first couple of days, each monkey would repeatedly climb up to look out and quickly slide back down. Within a couple of days, though, they gave up, sitting in the middle of the device and not moving. They became almost unresponsive. When they returned to their families, they didn't revert back to normal social behavior. It didn't matter what problems the monkey had prior to the experiment; both the abnormal monkeys and normal monkeys became despondent. Even the "best" monkeys from very stimulating and interactive families would succumb.

The apparatus was named "The Pit of Despair." It was felt that this learned helplessness resulted from a combination of feeling the loss of a good life reinforced by occasional glimpses of it. Within a half a week, every monkey spiraled downward. What was even more disturbing was that the monkeys did not spontaneously resolve their depression after being let out of the cage. Even actively treating the depression was not always successful.

Think of the promises held out by physical therapy, chiropractic adjustments, injections, acupuncture, vocational retraining, medications, traction, inversion tables, and finally surgery. How many times can your expectations be dashed before you lose hope?

## Life in the Abyss

Anger firmly holds you in one place. A metaphor for anger is how they restrain elephants in India. When the elephants are small, they are held in one place by tying or chaining one foot to a stake. When the elephant has turned into a huge adult, it will still be restrained by the same type of small stake. The animals have been programmed to think of the stake as something that cannot be pulled up. Anger is similar. You must be aware of the restraint.

Becoming socially isolated is another aspect of life in the Abyss. When I ask my patients about their social lives, they usually just shake their heads with a sad look. In addition to friends and family becoming tired of hearing you complain, your energy is drained by your body being bathed in stress hormones. You don't feel like being social. As you become more isolated, a higher percentage of your consciousness is spent experiencing pain and frustration. Your formerly productive life is consumed.

A 2003 study demonstrated that when volunteers were met with perceived social isolation, the same part of the brain lit up on a functional MRI as it did when they experienced physical pain.[11] The findings were consistent. This is yet another loop that is present with chronic pain: you become isolated and experience even more pain than before. Then the increased pain makes it less likely that you'll reach out to your friends and family. In fact, not only do patients not reach out, they often lash out at those they need for support, driving them away.

If you are in the Abyss, your family is also in the Abyss. Lashing out at loved ones has an effect on them and they don't deserve it. My abusive mother suffered from chronic pain. It was confusing for me to feel one moment like I had a mother who would do anything for her family and then, the next moment, watch her fly into a rage that could last for several days. From a young child's perspective, it was terrifying.

I read a book during my late teens that shed some light on my mother's behavior. It is a brilliant book by M. Scott Peck called *People of the Lie.*[12] He begins with a story of a twelve-year-old boy who had a near-psychotic break after he was given a .22-caliber rifle for Christmas. His parents were confused in that they felt that they were making a positive statement to him: he was entering his teen years and they trusted him enough to believe he could be responsible with a gun. The problem was that it was the same gun that his fifteen-year-old brother had used to commit suicide the prior Christmas. These parents, like my mother, were unaware of their child's needs.

Being unaware of another person's needs is the essence of abuse. If you are consumed by anger while trying to keep your head above water, you may well become fixated on your own needs and unable to view a situation through another person's eyes. How do you think your children or partner perceives your mood and actions? How do you think a five-year-old feels when you're exhibiting anger—maybe even rage—because you have once again been disappointed by the medical world, or beaten up by Workers' Comp? You may not think of your actions as abusive, but it is abuse.

## The Ultimate Modifier—Anger—Final Thoughts

Anger is the greatest obstacle to creating a healthy, pain-free life. It separates you from yourself, those closest to you, and life, and it is impossible to move forward until you are able to use strategies to process it and move forward. How victimized do you feel by your pain and the circumstances surrounding it? How angry are you that no one seems willing to listen to you, believe you, or care about your pain? How attached are you to your victim role? How willing are you to look at whether it's running your life?

The victim role is universal. The willingness to take an honest look at it is not. Asking yourself all the above questions will help you get closer to moving out of this role—and out of the Abyss. The only way out of it is through you. If you are not aware you're in it, you will remain there.

# SECTION 2:
# DOC PRINCIPLES

# CHAPTER 6

## Processing Stress

CONTRARY TO POPULAR BELIEF, STRESS IS NOT THE PRIMARY SOURCE of our unhappiness. Rather, it's our reaction to it that drains our energy. Why? Because stress causes negative thoughts. And despite the fact that, as it's been pointed out for many centuries, "you are not your thoughts," we usually identify with them because we feel the reaction caused by stress hormones. Thoughts are real and so is our physical reaction to them. But they are not our reality—unless we allow them to be.

I am defining a stressor as *any situation or circumstance that causes an automatic mental and physical survival reaction.* (Note that while the stressors I refer to in this chapter are difficult situations, positive events such as weddings, buying a new house, career changes, etc., are also stressors.)

It's difficult to consider not having an extreme reaction to certain stressful situations; for example, if your basic survival needs (shelter, food, and water) aren't met, or you are physically disabled. I do not want to minimize that level of suffering. Being free of pain is also a basic need.

When it comes to being in chronic pain, your reaction to stress will either magnify or diminish your body's physical response and suffering. Strategies to minimize your reactions and calm yourself will improve your quality of life.

## The Terrifying Triad

If you're reading this book, your life probably is not exactly as you'd like it to be. Your pain is significantly affecting your quality of life and you're not happy about it. The medical profession hasn't provided an adequate explanation for why you're in pain; you've been offered multiple treatments that initially raised your hopes for a better life, yet the treatments didn't result in any lasting relief. As the pain drags on and your expectations aren't met, you become more and more anxious and frustrated. You are trapped without any hope of escape. In addition, your nervous system is being pounded by pain impulses. It's an intersection of the neurological pathways of pain, anxiety, and anger—what I refer to as "the terrifying triad."

As discussed earlier, anxiety occurs when a basic human need such as air, food, or water isn't met. If this happens, we take action to meet the need and allay our anxiety. If we can't take action, anxiety escalates to anger.

To illustrate my point in clinic I ask my patients, "What would happen to your anxiety if you held your hand over a hot burner on a stove?"

"It would increase."

"What would be your response?"

"I would pull back my hand."

Then I ask, "What would happen to your anxiety if I took your arm and forced you to continue to hold your hand over the burner?" My patients' eyes roll in response to such an obvious question and they reply, "It would go up."

The next question results in a surprisingly wide range of answers. Patients are also slightly incredulous that I am asking them these questions. I lean forward and grab their arm and say, "I am serious. Picture me holding your arm and not letting you move it away from the hot burner. What would be your next response?" Most people state that they would become angry but I also hear, "I would panic," "I would punch you," and "I don't know." I wonder what the answer is telling me about this patient because many of the answers reflect helplessness and giving up.

When you are trapped by pain, it is analogous to being forced to hold your hand over the hot burner of a stove. There's no escape, no end point, and you have lost control. Over time, you will develop what Dr. John Sarno describes as rage.[1]

Pain, anxiety, and anger are linked, and these links infiltrate your life. So when you encounter other life stresses, such as having a difficult boss, being in a tumultuous relationship, or having trouble with finances, you will experience more pain. Why? Because these circuits are intertwined. Your brain works by association. It isn't imaginary or psychological; it's all connected and real.

My patients quickly become aware of the link between stress and pain. They see that when their stress reaches a certain level, there's consistently a corresponding increase in their pain. Sometimes it is so severe that I feel compelled to reorder diagnostic tests, which are usually unremarkable.

## Situational Stress

I have discovered with just minimal questioning that many (if not most) of my patients have incurred a major personal loss around the time that their pain flared up. The losses are often multiple, resulting in extreme feelings of stress and hopelessness. This does not even include the stress of pain.

One example was a woman in her sixties who had pain from a bone spur in her lower spine, causing sciatica. Historically I would quickly have signed her up for surgery but I have slowly learned the art of finding out what else is occurring in my patients' lives. Not only had she lost her job, her husband had left her, and her teenage son had been diagnosed with cancer. I told her, as I now tell all of my patients, that I will not perform elective spine surgery in the face of severe personal losses.

A patient's pain will frequently resolve once they have recovered (or have started recovering) from their loss, even in the presence of a significant structural problem. Indeed, her pain disappeared within about three months, after she worked through her losses.

I have become increasingly aware of the role of situational stresses in firing up pain in the distribution of pre-existing pathology. What has become obvious is that, while a given patient's pain might have begun a few months earlier, their lesion—such as a bone spur—may have been there for many years. Why is it flaring up now?

## "My Son Just Died"

George was a semi-retired banker who acted and looked about half his age. He was pleasant and talked freely about the pain down the side of his left leg, which had been a problem for about six months. It was worse when standing and walking, and immediately disappeared when he sat down. His MRI scan revealed that he had a bone spur pushing on his fifth lumbar nerve root out to the side of his spine. As his symptoms and history matched the abnormal anatomy, it seemed like an easy decision to offer him a one-level fusion. He was the ideal surgical candidate, as he was so motivated and physically fit.

I rarely make a surgical decision on the first visit, but George's situation appeared to be so straightforward that I decided to make an exception. He also wanted to proceed quickly, as he was frustrated by his limitations.

As I walked out the door to grab the pre-operative letter that describes the details of the fusion, he quietly said, "My son just died a few months ago." I immediately turned around and sat down with him. He said that his son had died from a massive heart attack. I let him know how sorry I was about his loss, and also told him that I was not comfortable with him making such a major decision in light of the situation. He agreed. I handed him the pre-op letter and asked him to return in a couple of weeks. I also gave him a copy of an earlier version of this book so he could gain an understanding of the various aspects of chronic pain. A week later he called and told me that he really wasn't into reading my book and just wanted to proceed with surgery. I asked him one more time just to glance through the book, as it does help with post-operative pain and rehab; and I signed him up for surgery.

George's wife accompanied him for his pre-operative appointment to coordinate the final details around the operation. I wanted be sure that we were on the same page regarding the severity of the pain and his understanding of the procedure. He said, "I am feeling better. I have read parts of your book and think that maybe I should work through some of the issues around my son's death." We had a long conversation about the effect this degree of trauma can cause. He asked me if I was okay with him delaying his surgery for a while.

I saw George a month later and he had no pain. He was fully active and had just re-joined the gym. I asked him what seemed to be the most helpful strategy in resolving his pain. He said he'd continued to read the book, which had built his level of awareness. Just understanding the links between anxiety, anger, trauma, and pain had helped him make sense of the different emotions he was trying to process. He was also now talking to his friends about his loss and they were offering a lot of support. His whole demeanor had changed and he was now more concerned about how the situation was affecting his wife. Several years later he still has no pain.

## Principles of Dealing with Stress

As discussed earlier in the book, I experienced chronic pain for about fifteen years. I feel strongly that much of my harsh experience could have been avoided if I hadn't made so many mistakes along the way. Learning these stress management strategies much earlier would have had a major impact in my life. Here are some of those principles:

- Stress management is a learned skill.
- Anxiety never gets better with time. Untreated, it gets worse.
- No human being escapes the relentless progression of anxiety— no one! Some are just better at disguising it for a while.
- Our coping patterns are programmed by our families and are typically not effective.
- Living a full life requires having a vision. As life beats us down, most of us lose that vision. It is critical to reconnect with that vision, in spite of the pain.
- The essence of dealing with stress is having awareness. This is the opposite of positive thinking, which breeds thought suppression. Awareness connects us to our thoughts and to the details of our environment.

Stress will always play a role in our lives; it's unavoidable. What's more, trying to avoid stress will become a major stressor in itself, causing your life to shrink.

## Two Aspects of Managing Stress

There are two aspects of dealing with stress. One is caring for yourself and building up your reserves, and the other is becoming aware of what drains your energy and plugging the drain.

Building up your energy reserves is the best way to cope with stress.

Some strategies include getting adequate sleep, exercising, spending time with friends and family, spending quiet time alone, and engaging in enjoyable activities. Getting organized and living within a budget are also helpful. These strategies are valuable, but there is a problem: coping with stress in this way is a rational attempt to deal with your unconscious brain. How does your unconscious brain play into it? Your body's reaction to stress is automatic. Your body treats any stress like a threat to your survival, generating an automatic hyper-vigilant reaction that will drain your energy.

That's why you not only have to build up your energy reserves to manage stress; you also have to plug the drain. How do you do so? By first understanding that the drain exists and is wide open. Anxiety-driven anger is the drain.

Picture your life as a bathtub. The water flowing through the faucet represents the enjoyable, rejuvenating parts of your life. Then visualize an unusually large drain that represents anger. If you're angry, that means the drain is wide open, and no matter how much water you pour into the tub, it will never fill up. It will be impossible to build up your energy reserves to the level you need to fully enjoy your life.

Or, picture trying to cross a river while rowing a boat with a hole in the bottom. The boat is slowly sinking, and you can't both bail and navigate. Even if it were possible, it would certainly detract from the enjoyment of the trip.

Now imagine running the bath water with the drain closed. You've learned how to process your frustrations and now you can relax into the tub and calm your senses. Likewise, the rowboat is no longer sinking, so you can enjoy the journey.

### *Having It All*
We intellectually know from the personal tragedies of high-profile stars that "having it all" does not ensure a happy and fulfilling life. Yet we

somehow think that if we just had what they did, we would be happier. It really does not work. In fact, having it all can make you feel worse.

I have watched this phenomenon for years in patients and friends who achieved and accomplished their dreams but who still had crippling anxiety. My first hint of this occurred when I was listening to a fifty-year-old entrepreneurial patient who had just sold his business for over forty million dollars. One would think he'd be ecstatic, but he was a mess. He completely broke down in my office, saying, "What am I going to do? I've been working on this project for over twenty years."

I was more than a little perplexed. After all, he'd accomplished his goals of building a successful business, acquiring possessions, having a great family, and enjoying life in a resort town. I wished that I had his problem! But I was missing something in this scenario—even though I was personally experiencing my own severe anxiety, I didn't make the connection that external factors cannot quiet the noise in your head. His relentless anxiety, which had its roots in a turbulent childhood, was destroying an incredible life.

I still didn't understand the terrible power of anxiety-driven anger, even after I began to spiral into the Abyss myself. In 1990, I had a great spine practice in a top orthopedic group, owned a beautiful house near the city, was enjoying my family, played basketball a couple of times of week, and was able to travel. I started experiencing panic attacks, and I had no idea what they were or why they were occurring. Little did I realize, I had begun descending into the Abyss.

What else did I need in my life to feel good? That was the problem. One of my dominant recurring thoughts after the panic attacks began was, "This is not working. I have everything I have ever worked for and I am miserable. Now what do I do?" I was truly desperate and that was just the first month of a fifteen-year free fall.

The people who often have the hardest time plugging the drain are the ones who are good at taking care of themselves, at least externally. That was me—I was pretty good at "filling the tub." There were lots of positive aspects of my life: I knew how to enjoy myself, I spent time with friends and family, I exercised. I did not even realize that there was a drain and certainly had no idea to plug it. It cost me at least fifteen years of a quality life. Material possessions and great life experiences are no match for anxiety-driven anger.

## Plugging the Drain?

The way that most of us are taught to plug the drain is to avoid complaining and think positive thoughts. This approach plays out in many destructive ways. My approach from early high school was to "think positive" and tell myself, "I can do this." A few friends of mine in college referred to me as "the brick." I could put up a wall around anything. I knew at the time that from their perspective, it was not entirely complimentary. However, I took it as somewhat of a perverse badge of honor.

During summer breaks from early high school and continuing through my medical training, I worked in heavy construction. I framed, poured, and finished concrete slabs, carried a hod, and did some finish work. One hot summer afternoon I was framing a large house in Napa Valley. I hadn't slept much. One of my personal challenges was to consistently sink a 16-penny nail with two swings of the hammer and occasionally one. I was bent over, holding a stud against the floor plate and took a full swing with my 28-ounce framing hammer. The hammer glanced off an upright piece of plastic plumbing and landed squarely on my left thumb. The pain was so intense that I almost passed out. I stood up, looked at my mangled thumb, wrapped it up in a rag, and went back to work without a word. My boss, who'd been standing just ten feet away, thought I was out of my mind.

I later learned that being tough, however, doesn't yield a full and satisfying life. Neither does positive thinking. Toughness is actually a variant of positive thinking, and there are prices to pay for both. Being tough and/ or positive is like pushing a rock up an endless hill.

My toughness and positive thinking eventually caught up with me. In 1988, I started going into a long period of burnout and depression. Later, I began to have severe anxiety reactions that, per above, progressed into panic attacks. By 1997, I had developed an obsessive-compulsive disorder, and within a few years I was seriously suicidal. I didn't survive the ordeal because I had a ray of hope; my darkness was complete. Only my ties with my family and friends pulled me through.

### *Really* Plugging the Drain

The essence of plugging the drain is to learn to separate yourself and your reaction from the stressful event. It's not the actual situation that drains your energy; it's your response, along with stress hormones.

The first step is to recognize your automatic reaction to adversity, which will always be an adrenaline survival response. Then you must create space between yourself and the stressor in order to substitute a better response. The sequence is awareness, separation, and reprogramming. Creating distance from and learning to live with adversity instead of fighting it is what plugs the drain.

Let's look at a stressful scenario and examine how a reaction impacts the event. Imagine a situation wherein your teenage son came home well after his curfew. As you confront him, he talks back, rejecting your authority and disrespecting you. Predictably and understandably, you become angry.

The stressor is your child coming in late and then responding aggressively when confronted. The situation, in and of itself, is not an energy drain. After all, you weren't physically harmed. Rather, it's your angry reaction that drains your energy and brings you down. If you identify with your reaction and you are the angry parent, then it all ends up feeling like one ugly event. By taking a step back in this setup and developing an awareness of the various parts of the interaction, you can more effectively deal with it.

As the adult, a better response would have been to avoid engaging in a conversation while you were upset, especially late at night. By waiting until morning, you could have defused your response and then talked things over in a civil manner. Have you ever noticed that an issue rarely gets solved when one or both parties are upset? Handling a situation poorly has fallout that can carry over into other aspects of your relationship for days, weeks, months, or even years. Instead of putting your relationship with a loved one at risk, take a time out.

Another example I frequently use in clinic involves driving. I ask my patient to imagine sitting in a long line of cars waiting to exit the freeway, and watching another car zoom ahead and cut into the front of the line. Then I ask, "You might get upset but what's the problem? No one was hurt. What exactly ruined your day? Was it the situation or your reaction?" If you drive, it's impossible to avoid interacting with bad drivers. You can't control that. So why would you give someone you feel is inconsiderate the power to upset you?

In both of these stressful situations—the curfew confrontation and the driving—it's important to stop and create an *awareness* of each part of the circumstances. You can do this by visualizing how you must appear while you are upset. It's not going to be a pleasant sight. Then consider how your reaction interfered with your quality of life or negatively impacted your relationships. Is this the way you want to continue to live your life? How would you feel about your child acting the way you have? There is no right answer, but just considering the issues slows down your mind and you now have a choice about how you might react in the future.

Anxiety and anger are not who you are. They are automatic survival reactions. They separate you from your value system and how you choose to live your life. Until you can separate these reactions from your core identity, the drain in the tub will remain wide open. Become aware of the drain and how it's affecting you, and learn the methods to plug it. Specific ways to accomplish this will be presented throughout the rest of the book.

## The Effect of Stress on Pain

Learning how to effectively process stress will decrease your pain. When my patients start the DOC process, they all quickly see the connection between their levels of stress and pain. As their stress decreases, so does their pain. And then, as they feel better, they often have the urge to rid themselves completely of stress and pain. When adversity inevitably hits, as it does in all our lives, they become upset. But this project is not about being endlessly happy. It's about full engagement, with both joy and pain. Both happen.

No one is asking you to be happy when you have suffered a loss or have been treated badly. This process is about nurturing connected and engaged thinking based on awareness—awareness of the stress and your reaction to it. When things are bad, you may feel worse, but when you have healed, you are also able to really enjoy the good times.

When you *are* stressed, it's important to allow yourself to feel the full impact of it. Then you can process it more rapidly and not remain in the hole. Eventually you will dive into the Abyss less often and emerge more quickly.

As you go through the DOC process, you will also learn to live with anxiety and anger, and unconsciously your body will have less of a stress response. It is one of the paradoxes of this process that the more comfortable you are in experiencing negative emotions, the less power they will have, and the less often they will occur.

Dr. Fred Luskin is a Stanford psychologist and author of *Forgive for Good.*[3] During a seminar we were doing together, he had everyone lie on the floor with our eyes closed. He asked us to visualize someone we were close to and cared for and experience what that felt like. He then instructed us to consider someone we despised and still hold on to the feelings of peace and love. I don't think any of it succeeded on this first try, but you get the idea. You can train your body to keep from reacting physiologically to adversity.

As you become more aware of your reaction to stress and how to separate from it, your pain will predictably decrease. When I encounter patients who cannot seem to pull out of their pain pathways, it is almost always centered around holding onto deep anger. Let it go. You are the only one who is suffering. As Oscar Wilde said, "Always forgive your enemies; nothing annoys them so much."

## Processing Stress—Final Thoughts

One evening, while watching the news, I heard a report on the progress of Hurricane Gustav as it approached New Orleans. As I watched the satellite and radar pictures, a metaphor evolved in my mind. The whirling wind represented my racing thoughts, and the further away I was from my "center," the greater impact these thoughts were having on the quality of my day. Historically, I have attempted to slow down or suppress these thoughts. I wasted a lot of energy, and as I became drained, the thoughts would race even faster.

The wind can also represent life circumstances. We spend a lot of time attempting to control our circumstances in order to allay our anxiety and be happier, but the majority of situations in life are not controllable. The key with both racing thoughts and our life circumstances is to use tools to pull ourselves into the center. You cannot stop a hurricane, and once you quit wasting your efforts trying, your energy levels will soar.

# CHAPTER 7

# Awareness

AWARENESS IS THE FIRST AND NECESSARY STEP on your journey to health, as what you're not aware of can and will control you. If you're unaware of the depth of your anger and anxiety, you will be ruled by these emotions, day in and day out.

## Defining Awareness

Awareness is seeing the world as it actually is—not your interpretation of it. Pure awareness is almost impossible in the human experience; we look at life through our preprogrammed perceptions of reality that start to develop at birth. But the closer we can come to pure awareness, the more functional we can be as human beings. Awareness is the key to developing meaningful relationships; in a one-on-one encounter, the greater your capacity to see a situation through the other person's eyes, the greater chance of developing intimacy.

Intellectually, we understand the importance of awareness, and yet most of us continue to struggle with gaining true awareness. Why is that? Consider the following:

- Anxiety clouds awareness, but we are often not aware of our anxiety until it becomes disruptive.
- Anger covers up the feeling of anxiety, making it yet more difficult to be aware.
- The adrenaline that is released with anger decreases the blood flow to the frontal lobes of your brain. You cannot think clearly.

Chronic pain is resolvable if you become aware of its nature, your reactions to it, and the relevant variables that affect your perception of it. The first step in becoming aware is understanding when you are *not* aware.

### Becoming Aware of Unawareness

As I look back on my life journey, one of the most disturbing aspects is to realize the extent of my unawareness.

I was raised in a difficult family environment and by my eighteenth birthday, I had lived in twelve different houses. At age fifteen, I decided that I'd had enough of all the chaos and began to build my own life and persona. I worked hard at developing my identity and moved at warp speed for over twenty years. I was idealistic and thought I was a great student, and then a great husband, father, and doctor. The problem, in retrospect, was that I was connected to my identity—how I wanted to see myself and how others saw me—instead of to my true self. No one picked up on it, including me.

In my mind I was always right and could not figure out why people did not listen to my "wisdom" more carefully. I wasn't a good listener, myself, but I was unaware of this fact. I recall that someone once referred to my "obsessive nature." I didn't have a clue what they were talking about. I didn't know what the word really meant, but whatever sense I had of it, I was certain it didn't apply to me.

I was able to outwardly perform my "roles" in life very well until I experienced a panic attack out of the blue at age thirty-seven. My identity started to fall apart and then fifteen years of chronic pain stripped away the rest of my facade.

That period of my life didn't need to be that difficult. It was largely due to my unawareness. How can you tap into your unawareness? One way is to look for cues in certain behaviors and attitudes that may mean you're out of touch with how you're feeling. Some examples:

- Having a rigid opinion about almost anything: religion, politics, someone's character, etc.
- Being told you're stubborn or not listening
- Interrupting someone to offer an opinion before you've heard theirs in total
- Being "right"
- Consistently thinking about something besides what you're doing
- Judging yourself or others negatively or positively
  - Being persistently critical of your spouse, partner, and/or children
  - Giving unsolicited advice
- Feeling anxious or angry
- Thinking you're wiser than your children
- Acting on impulse

The list is endless. The first fifty years of my life, most if not all of the above applied to me, and yet I had no insight into my unawareness; if I started to feel any negative emotions, I quickly suppressed them. The list still applies to me, although my tools to deal with my unawareness have evolved. You will initially always view the world through your past experiences and learning. Dropping the filter of your perspective is a life-time task.

If you noticed some of the above behaviors or attitudes in yourself, it's probably time to take a step back and begin to work on seeing the world through other peoples' eyes. I still use these cues daily, as awareness is a minute-by-minute experience.

One of these cues, self-judgment, was a big part of my life and a major sign that I was unaware of my own patterns. It happened during my period of severe burnout, which occurred concurrently to my chronic pain. During that era, I had endless self-doubts and negative judgments about almost every aspect of my life. A severe case of perfectionism didn't help the situation. I often thought how much better it would be if I could judge myself positively with as much fervor.

I did turn my life around, and I've been able to help many people by drawing on the lessons I learned in barely surviving a severe depression. My practice has grown and I have an excellent reputation. I enjoy my family and friends. It's great to enjoy the fruits of one's labors. However, as soon as I go into a mode of "what a compassionate guy I am" or "what a great surgeon I am," it takes me right down. Any effort on my part to spin my life in a positive way to others drains me of the energy I need to be creative and also distracts me from being aware of what's occurring right in front of me. For me, it turns out that positive self-judgment is just as disruptive as negative self-judgment. It's still judgment. Once you have placed a label on anyone or anything, you can no longer see clearly.

Another clue, not listening, is one that I discovered with others' help. It became readily apparent while attending a parents' seminar for my stepdaughter's school, Hyde, in Bath, Maine. The seminars reflect the school's philosophy that knowledge, in and of itself, does not prepare you adequately for a successful life; the student's character should be the primary focus. Family members attend seminars three times a year because Hyde recognizes that much of everyone's character is shaped by interactions with parents and siblings.

I was initially quite cynical about the whole idea of attending these seminars. I'd already done a lot of work on myself and wasn't sure what else I could learn. In these group sessions, I would often spend a lot of time and effort "sharing my wisdom." I had learned a lot and did have a lot to offer. However, as others pointed out, it's difficult to learn with your mouth open.

I will preface this story by saying that I had always considered myself to be a good listener; it was one of my major personal identities. My wife, historically, has not always agreed with that viewpoint. Of course, I didn't listen to her.

In one exercise, we had to write down a characteristic that we thought another parent could work on. We could write to two parents and not include our names. (This is one of those games that you are not anxious to win.) Most parents received one or two slips of paper. I received twelve (out of eighteen) that all said the same thing: "David, you don't know how to listen."

That was a difficult moment for me. I found it hard not to become defensive, but on the other hand, how could I disagree with twelve people? I came to accept that they were right, especially in retrospect. It was a trait that I truly could not see. I had to trust a group of people who I knew did not have an agenda and had my best interests at heart. I came to realize how "not listening" had interfered with my general awareness. It's one of the central tenets of awareness: you cannot be aware if you cannot listen.

The definition of awareness that resonates most with me is "being fully present in the moment." In other words, I'm most aware when I'm able to listen, feel, and observe multiple cues and then appropriately respond to the person or situation. It requires stillness and silence in one's head.

## Unawareness and Abuse

Very few people who abuse others do so intentionally. They are usually consumed with anxiety-driven anger and are simply unaware of anyone else's needs. Their needs supersede all others' needs.

I had a patient years ago who was personable and rational when in my office. He was also addicted to narcotics, and the difficulties started when I began to wean him off of them. He eventually threatened to kill me when I refused to give him medications at the level he wanted. We had to call the police and put our clinic under guard. He also assaulted his grandmother for money to obtain drugs. His addiction had consumed him to the point where he could see only his own needs.

Not until I had a long conversation with my father about my mother's abusiveness did I become aware of how strongly chronic pain is connected to abuse. Even though I saw medications all over the house while growing up, I hadn't comprehended that she suffered from chronic pain. Between her rages, she was an incredibly committed mother and had a lot of remorse after every episode of her abusive behavior. I'm now aware of the link between abuse and pain, and am direct with my patients about this problem.

Breaking through patients' unawareness of their abusive behavior is extremely difficult because they don't recognize their anger and don't see their actions toward those close to them as abusive. They think that they're just expressing their legitimate frustrations. Becoming aware that your behavior might be considered abusive is tough. It's not how you'd like others to perceive you, and certainly not how you'd like to perceive yourself.

Often people who are abusive make up for it by being pillars of the community or church. They may hold an elevated position. Maybe they are active in a charity. A patient of mine who was a local business leader, prominent in local politics, and vocal about how others should live their lives, perpetrated one of the worst sexual abuse cases I have encountered. One of the disguises of anger is "being right" or "living life with conviction." Eventually, it came to light that he had been sleeping with his daughter for many years. When it was revealed about twenty years later, his remorse was extreme. In his mind he had been a very committed father.

Verbal abuse is extremely common but recognized by few. It can be just as devastating as any other type of abuse, though. Being regularly critical is the essence of it, but it's inherent in other behaviors as well: withholding words of affection, being silent, or not saying anything to actively help family members enjoy their day. Also, whenever you blame someone for creating your unhappiness and let them know it, you're probably being verbally abusive. *You are the only one responsible for your happiness*—end of story. The problem is very clearly outlined in Patricia Evans's book, *Verbal Abuse: Survivors Speak Out.*[1]

If you're suffering from chronic pain, there is a significant chance you're being abusive to those close to you. Ask them. I will request that my patients pose that question to their family and invariably they return for the next office visit visibly shaken up.

To improve your relationship with your family, my advice is to refrain from giving any advice to anyone for a month and to focus, instead, on listening. Talk with family members about creating a paradigm shift. It can be difficult to do this but my patients who've tried it say that it works, and they find the changes in their family dynamic gratifying. Don't make people you care about into targets of your frustrations.

It also works the other way around. If you are living with someone in chronic pain, there is a high probability that you're allowing yourself to be abused. Becoming aware of this possibility is critical before you can address the problem. The key question is, "Why would you allow yourself to be treated like this by anyone—especially your family?"

## The Four Levels of Awareness

I have discovered that observing myself go in and out of awareness is the essence of becoming aware. I consider awareness from four perspectives:

- Environmental
- Emotional
- Judgement and storytelling
- Ingrained patterns

### *Environmental Awareness*

Environmental awareness is becoming aware of as much detail as possible about what is right in front of you. The most effective method for accomplishing this is using what I call "active meditation," which is an abbreviated form of mindfulness. This practice involves briefly placing your attention on sensations. Any one will do—taste, feel, sound, pressure, etc. There are three steps and it just takes five to ten seconds.[2] Here are the steps:

1. Relax: I often begin by relaxing my shoulders; you can use any body part. Or I take a deep breath.
2. Stabilize: just feel the body part you relaxed for a few seconds before going to Step 3.
3. Focus on one sensation: taste, feel, sound, pressure, etc. Feel the vividness of the sensation increase.

Active meditation accomplishes several things. As you relax, your body will begin to secrete less adrenaline. When you give attention to a given sensation, your nervous system shifts off the pain circuits.

Active meditation becomes more automatic with practice. The pain pathways will eventually become weaker and the other pathways—the ones attached to the sense you're focused on—will become stronger. Eventually, you will get to a tipping point and become pain-free.

One metaphor that comes to mind is diverting a large river into another channel. Initially, very little water will flow through the new riverbed but with continued excavation the flow will increase. Eventually, just the force of the water will create a new river. The old riverbed is still there (it's permanent) but it fills in and becomes smaller.

I've found environmental awareness to be very helpful, but note that it can work in the opposite direction and markedly *increase*, instead of *decrease*, your pain. If much of your attention is focused on your discomfort, your nervous system will progressively feel more pain.

This happened with a friend of mine, who had a simple procedure on his leg. He was usually the type of person who wouldn't have thought much about it, but he also had experienced some recent losses and was more reactive than usual. He monitored every sensation in his leg and began to use a cane. Within six weeks, his lower leg pain was intolerable. He eventually developed a chronic pain syndrome requiring medications. There is little question in my mind that his pain would have resolved within a week, had this minimal procedure been performed during a less chaotic phase of his life. This instance demonstrates how quickly your brain adapts to where you choose to place your attention.

What I like about active meditation is that it's done in real time while you are fully engaged in living life. Endless stresses barrage us and this technique quickly allows you to stay calm. Eventually, you will be able handle more stress than you could ever imagine.

I am also a proponent of traditional meditation practices. It involves using a number of methods to connect fully with the present moment through sensations. One technique is to focus only on your breath, becoming aware of as many aspects of your breathing as you can. Various thoughts will enter your mind, and you will watch them come and go. The goal is not to ignore these thoughts, but to learn to not react to them. This is the process of separation. After the momentary distraction, you gently pull yourself back to your breathing as quickly as possible.

Traditional meditation isn't usually done in the context of your daily life, but it does assist in resetting and calming your baseline state, and is therefore a great complement to active meditation.

Environmental awareness is the baseline awareness that engages me in the present moment regardless of the circumstances. It's the anchor point upon which to build the other levels of awareness.

## Full Environmental Immersion

In my opinion, being completely immersed in an activity you are passionate about is the closest way to achieve complete environmental awareness. I will never forget an encounter I had with a patient named Fred, who was about fifty and had been suffering from total body pain for over thirty years. He had been bounced around the medical system and was not that happy to see me.

Fred was extremely skilled at building beautiful motorcycles. He showed me some pictures of his choppers, which were stunning. Suddenly he leaned over and said to me, "I am never in pain when I am in my shop." Back then I could not fathom how that was possible. Now that I understand the neurological basis of chronic pain it makes perfect sense. When you are engaging your pleasure pathways, you are disengaged from the pain circuits.

### *Emotional Awareness*

Connecting with your emotions and becoming aware of your reactivity is particularly critical. If your emotions are out of control, they will inflame your pain. Ideally, we'd all be aware of our emotional state at any given moment, but there are several obstacles. First, we don't start from a neutral position, but rather live in our own frame of reference. If, for instance, you were raised in an anxiety-ridden, abusive household, anxiety would be your normal emotional state in adulthood. Until your anxiety overwhelmed you, it would be hard to know how much it was driving your normal behavior. Second, none of us likes to experience negative emotions, so we tend to automatically deny or suppress them rather than come to terms with them. Third, when you are angry, all awareness is obliterated and you cannot connect with any emotions. Anger is the antithesis of awareness.

So how do we become more emotionally aware? The first step is to allow yourself to feel anything and everything. This includes anxiety. Anxiety represents being vulnerable to danger and we are programmed to avoid this feeling at all costs. Once you are able to feel this level of emotion you can feel a full range of emotions. This is a learned skill that cannot be accomplished intellectually. It involves actually feeling the uncomfortable sensations and remaining relaxed.

Anger is the biggest block to feeling vulnerable. Anger represents power, which completely blocks the ability to feel vulnerable. We like power and we hate feeling helpless. No one willingly wants to give up anger.

What makes this scenario even more confusing is that when we're angry, we want to blame someone or something. We don't realize that our anger response is a result of being triggered by a circumstance. We are responsible for our own anger even though it sometimes feels like someone else's fault. This is a challenge to comprehend—in fact, it's the most difficult part of understanding anger and dealing with it.

One book that I've found helpful in understanding anger is *The Way to Love* by Anthony deMello.[3] He teaches that you must learn to thank your enemy because they are a window into who you really are. He defines love as awareness.

•••••

Robert Hoffman (co-developer of the Hoffman Process) used the psychological term "transference" for the phenomenon of being triggered.[4] Here is Hoffman's definition of transference:

> Transference distorts relationships. Transference is reacting to and perceiving another person as if they are the mother and father from our childhood. Usually we are not aware that we are doing it. We believe we are really seeing that other person in the present moment. When we are in transference with another person, we often feel a certainty that we know who they are. We usually feel we know what they are feeling and thinking, what their intentions are, and what we can and cannot expect from them.
>
> When we are in negative transference (a much more common occurrence for most of us), we feel the energy of certainty about the other person's wrongness. At times, the transference is triggered by an actual behavior of the other person. They don't look us in the eye, or they do. They criticize our work. They are sarcastic or late or forget to do something. Many times the transference is triggered only by our perception that they did something wrong and our interpretation of what that means. We go into a vicious cycle within ourselves. We feel that another person has done something wrong to us. We think we know all about them, what they did, and what they will do, think, and feel. They are powerful—we give them the power to affect our lives—and we are powerless. We often feel little, like a child in the face of a negative parent. That's where we went internally even if we do not recognize it consciously.
>
> Actually we have the power, if we choose to use it, to change the dynamic, to stop reacting. The actions of others trigger us because we have the patterns in us.

The Hoffman Process taught me that no one can make you angry; you have a choice every time your anger button is pushed. The problem is that it doesn't *feel* like you have a choice because the transference response is so fast and powerful. It gives you a strong conviction of your "rightness."

Sudden action is often taken while under the spell of transference; it's a dangerous situation.

If you can't connect with your true emotional state, you will not be able to embark on a journey of self-discovery. You can't see who you really are unless you commit to stepping outside of your mind and looking at yourself from a different perspective. Ask yourself these questions: "Am I open?" "Am I coachable?" "Can I really listen and feel?" This is a starting point. Beyond that, active meditation is remarkably effective for self-discovery, as are the writing exercises I advocate in this book. Then there's external help—it's impossible to evolve without it. There are self-help books, counseling, meditation, seminars, retreats, and more. Once you get in touch with what's going on in your mind, you can go on a very powerful journey.

Why don't more people pursue a path of self-discovery? It may be because, in our culture, most of us spend a lot of emotional energy trying to look good to people around us as well as to ourselves. Truly connecting with our emotions is an act of humility; it's also extremely rewarding, and it makes life much easier in the end.

### *Judgment and Storytelling*

A third level of awareness revolves around judgment and storytelling. On this level, you create a "story" or a judgment about yourself, another person, or situation that tends to be rough and inflexible.

The brain is programmed to look for danger and will first focus on negative judgments. David Burns, in his book *Feeling Good*[5,] categorized these cognitive distortions into "ten errors in thinking." When we make these errors, we create stories out of circumstances that are often non-events. Burns calls these negative thoughts "ANTS," which stands for "automatic negative thoughts."

For example, imagine someone at work walked by you and didn't acknowledge you. You might think they're upset with you about a situation that occurred the day before. The error in thinking in this case would be "mind reading." You can't read other people's minds; it's possible that the person had just received some bad news and wasn't engaging with anyone.

Then there is the error of "labeling." For example, a frequently late spouse becomes "inconsiderate." A forgetful teenager becomes "irresponsible." By labeling, especially negative labeling, you can no longer see them because you are only projecting your version of reality onto them. You have limited your capacity to enjoy being with them.

What about the labels we have for ourselves? You knock something over and call yourself "clumsy." In addition to labeling, this error falls under "should" thinking. If a lover breaks up with you, then you're "unlovable." Rehashing these critical judgments in our minds turns them into deeply embedded stories.

Such stories are much harder to move on from than single judgments. Once a judgment sets into a story, you tend to lose all perspective. Over time, faulty thinking can become your reality. Labeling groups of people is also the basis of societal atrocities. It's important to recognize when an error in thinking becomes a story because much of our lives tend to be run on stories that have little to do with reality.

To better understand the story concept, consider common situations where the brain focuses on a self-perceived flaw that is not physically painful. It might be your height, weight, the shape of your body, or even an individual body part. Or it might be some particular quality, such as a lack of intelligence, athletic skill, musical talent, etc. Thinking about it over and over snares you in a destructive cycle of spinning neural circuits. Not thinking about it makes it even worse. For example, many years ago, I had a patient with neck pain who was absolutely convinced that he was "stupid." His self-labeling wasn't rational, as he was clearly a bright guy. He eventually developed a significant chronic burning sensation around his mouth without a physical cause.

Something similar happens in the entertainment industry, where performers commonly focus only on their negative reviews. My wife, who is a tap dancer, has seen this in her profession for years. She pointed out to me that a performer might have ninety-nine positive reviews but will fixate on the one that's negative. In fact, it's a common saying that "you're only as good as your worst critic."

Another common, perhaps universal, phenomenon is focusing on a spouse's or partner's negative trait or traits. The other person usually has innumerable positive qualities that are forgotten in the face of the flaw. Over time the "story" can become so strong it can break apart an otherwise great relationship.

What's curious to me is why the human brain does not become equally fixated on positive traits. Reconsidering Wegner's white bears experiment[6], maybe it's because we don't suppress positive thoughts. As proven in his experiment, fixation goes hand in hand with suppression.

## "I Didn't Want This Car"

When I think of judgment and storytelling, one particular event from my own life comes to mind. It shows how creating stories has the power to disrupt your peace of mind and detract from your enjoyment of life.

One Memorial Day weekend, my wife and I were taking my father for a ride up to beautiful Point Reyes on the coast north of San Francisco. About twenty minutes into our trip, I noticed that the car's low-tire-pressure light had come on. It was a brand new car with less than a thousand miles on it, so I thought it was probably just a malfunctioning light. I wasn't convinced that we'd made the correct decision to buy this car in the first place—it was more expensive than I was comfortable with—so I was more than a little frustrated that the light had a glitch.

I stopped to put some air in the tire, just in case, and then kept driving for another forty-five minutes. As we approached Point Reyes in the early afternoon, however, we realized that the tire was really low, so I pulled over to change it. But when I opened the trunk, there was no spare. The story in my head was starting to ramp up as I wondered in frustration why a new car wouldn't have a spare. I called the car company's roadside assistance line and they told me these new cars had "run-flat" tires that should be good for 150 miles at a maximum of fifty miles per hour. I felt a little insecure about that plan. We were a long way from the last large town we'd passed, and I thought that we should turn back. My wife thought that since my father rarely made it to visit, we should go out to dinner. So we headed toward a restaurant on the coast. About three miles down the road the tire exploded.

It was now about four o'clock in the afternoon on Memorial Day and we were miles from any town. Our only option was to get towed back courtesy of AAA. It was hard for me to process the fact that I had to get my new car towed for a flat tire. The tow-truck driver showed up to take us to the service station and let the three of us ride in the cab with my wife sitting on my lap. She started to complain about the bumpiness of the ride, which I found a little annoying. "I'm the one on the bottom," I thought. She wanted to have dinner in San Rafael and take a taxi home. I started to grind my teeth to keep my mouth shut.

This is how the afternoon had unfolded for me. Starting with the low tire, I'd made a decision to enjoy my time with my family in spite of the problem. I took note of my frustrations and concentrated on listening to the conversation and staying involved in the day. I was successful for a while—until the tire blew up. Then my anger began to bubble. I became aware that in spite of everything I'd learned about dealing with stress, I was greatly magnifying the problem with the thoughts in my head. I was thinking things like, "I can't believe I got talked into buying this car," "My wife made me buy it," "It's me at the bottom of this pile; why are you the one complaining?" and "The tow-truck driver must think we're out of our minds."

Although there might have been some truth in the things I was telling myself, I recognized that it wasn't helping us get through the situation. Nonetheless, I wasn't able to minimize my suffering through the stress relief techniques that had helped in the past, which was frustrating. I tried to talk myself out of it: "I know better. I can't control any of these variables right now, so let it go. I know how to do this." But it didn't work.

Then I began to go really dark with thoughts like, "How can I be married to this woman?" I began to notice how irrational and big these thoughts had become. It felt like a bomb had exploded. My misery was way out of proportion to the situation.

In this instance, I was guilty of multiple errors in thinking. They came in the form of labeling—for instance, "My wife is irresponsible"; and catastrophizing—"Why did we get married?" Through it all, I negated her many positive qualities. To cite one, she's great at keeping things light, no matter what the problem, and unlike me, she was able to keep her cool throughout the day.

I would usually have remained in this agitated state of mind for days with some carryover lasting for weeks. I wouldn't have been able to separate my wife's actions from my thoughts and realize that the problem wasn't her; it was my reaction to the situation. It was a major step for me to become aware of how out of proportion the story in my head had become. This degree of awareness really changed the game for me.

Eventually, we did get towed home. We went out to dinner. I practiced my own negative writing that evening. I still love my wife. I learned yet another lesson in humility.

### Ingrained Patterns

We all have ingrained patterns of behavior and thinking, which we develop over a lifetime of exposure to our environment. Our brain is hard-wired during our formative years and certain situations will elicit a predictable response. We don't recognize or feel these patterns; it's just what we do. It's behavior that sits under many layers of defenses and has to be dug out by each person. These ingrained habits and actions are much more obvious to our spouses and immediate family than they are to us; we can only get in touch with them through active work, like counseling, seminars, psychotherapy, self-reflection, and spousal feedback, for example. This lack of awareness is a huge problem in that, again, what you are not aware of will control you. Without becoming aware you will spend your entire life projecting your preprogrammed view of the world onto others.

I didn't realize the extent of my own unawareness until I was at a Hyde parents' seminar one weekend. The week before, my regional West Coast Hyde group had worked me over about issues with my son that I hadn't seen very clearly. I was not in a great mood. I was a little negative and had decided I would not contribute much to the group. What I didn't realize was that, as a result, I would end up actually listening.

I watched one father try to be the perfect Hyde seminar parent. He was a great, well-intentioned guy, but these very qualities were clearly blocking him from connecting with his son. I realized how often I had played that role in my own life.

One of the exercises was to write a final letter to myself about my core values. I decided to open up my mind a little more and asked myself the question, "If I'm so enlightened, why am I such a workaholic?" During this session, a story kept popping into my head from when I was a first-year orthopedic resident in Honolulu, Hawaii. About three months into my training, I overheard one of the other residents talking about admitting a patient with severe back pain who also had an anxiety disorder. I asked him, "What do you mean by anxiety disorder?" I had no idea what anxiety was; I had to look it up in a textbook.

Eventually, I developed a severe anxiety disorder. As I sat in the Hyde seminar room looking back, I couldn't figure out how I could have gone through college, medical school, and two years of internal medicine residency and not have had a clue about the nature of anxiety. Obviously, I'd encountered many anxiety-provoking situations.

That afternoon a bomb went off in my head. Anxiety, in fact, was all that I knew. I'd been raised in an abusive household, never knowing when my mother would explode. She was, at some level, experiencing rage most of the time. Fear was the basis of all of my behavior going forward. Most of my energy as a child was spent either trying not to set my mother off or calming her down. Most of my energy in adulthood was spent in avoiding unpleasant emotions: I dealt with anger by suppressing it and I addressed anxiety by staying distracted, mostly by my work.

It is, by definition, not possible to recognize your own ingrained patterns without being open to outside input or having the desire to develop self-awareness. Usually it takes some type of interaction with another person in an individual or group setting. Hyde set up a structure for me to realize my patterns. The didactic part of it was critical, but my paradigm shift would not have occurred without the support of the people in that room. They were instrumental in permanently changing my life.

## Putting the Awareness Model to Work

We work at becoming better and happier people. But the marketing world keeps reminding us that we haven't met our potential and holds up endless images of perfection to reinforce that idea. We're led to believe that we need a better appearance, more friends, a longer list of accomplishments, more public recognition, greater power, and on and on. The message is, "If I had more (or less) of 'X,' I would be a happier person." (The list includes less pain.) We are programmed into being defined by external factors. It's important to understand this impact from all levels of awareness.

If you're waiting for more wisdom, more money, a nicer spouse, better-behaved kids, or less pain before you can fully engage in your life, you'll be waiting forever. It's illogical to think that all the variables in our lives will align so well that we'll have perfect fulfillment. And even if it could happen, how long do you think it would last? Think how much energy we spend trying to control so much.

I remind my patients that there is no goal to the DOC (Define your Own Care) project. A few years ago, I realized that there is an endless number of ways to work on myself through the DOC process. That meant that there was no endpoint and the "goal" of the project was merely to enjoy one's day using whatever skills one possesses, no matter what the current set of circumstances, including pain levels. All levels of awareness come into play with this approach.

Here's how I put the awareness model to work: first, anytime I am anxious or angry, I remind myself that I am in a preprogrammed reactive pattern—a survival response. That allows me to become aware of my emotions and the pattern. Then I use environmental awareness to assess all the variables that may have triggered me. Active meditation is part of this process and I can usually calm down relatively quickly. I have an endless number of "stories" and judgments of those around me and become aware how I am projecting my negative self-talk on to others. When the dust has settled, I contemplate how I must have appeared to the person I was upset at and I don't like it. This is the phase where I think about my overall behavior and realize that many of my ingrained behaviors and belief systems are destructive.

Finally, I make a decision to enjoy the rest of my day, period. I make deliberate choices to be kind and patient with myself and others; keep my perspective and remain grateful; and to take time to appreciate any good things that come my way, such as a warm greeting from a partner or friend, or a good meal. There are many other examples, but you get the idea.

It sounds like this process would take a while but it occurs in only a few seconds. It can be simplified into becoming aware and calming down. A metaphor that I keep in mind is one I learned from a small book on Taoism.[7] Picture a stork quietly standing on one leg at the edge of a pond. When a fish swims by it reaches down and grabs its next meal. It doesn't fly around aimlessly looking for food. The message is that you can deal with what is in front of you and then let the rest go. You have to become aware of what you have no control over.

## An Awareness Mantra

One of most aware people I've ever met was an eighty-year-old patient whose sense of peace and calm was striking. He was a light. I used to see him when he worked as a volunteer at my hospital and he was always open and friendly. He became my patient when he developed sciatica from a bone spur. As I worked with him, I was impressed by how he handled the pain and adversity. I finally asked him why he was so happy. He was initially hesitant in responding but two weeks later he sent me an email with what he thought were the key ingredients to enjoying his life.

I am whole and powerful.
I am loving and harmonious.
I am forgiving and happy. I am at peace.

I thought this mantra was great but it just wouldn't stick with me. About a year later, the light came on during a disagreement with my one of my partners. I was certainly not at peace. I was angry and couldn't let it go. I was also frustrated with myself because, intellectually, I knew I had to let it go. After all, I write about and teach these concepts. Suddenly, I understood the connections between the words.

- If you are whole, you don't have to expend energy filling gaps. The result is power to live your life.
- Love is often described as absence of fear. Harmony is the result.[8]
- It's impossible to be happy without forgiveness.
- You won't be at peace without all of the above.

Using awareness, I have learned to work backwards through this mantra. Whenever I am not at peace, I ask myself, "Am I not being forgiving and therefore unhappy?" "Am I not being loving and therefore out of harmony?" "What is making me feel that I'm not whole?" Usually I can see what is disrupting my peace of mind.

Most of my chronic pain patients are not at peace. One reason is lack of forgiveness, which is difficult in the context of chronic pain.

One of my patients had had pain throughout her whole body for over five years. I was struck by the intensity of her rage. She'd suffered several major fractures, including a broken pelvis in a car accident. All of the fractures had healed so there was not a surgical solution for her pain. She was upset and openly frustrated with me. Then I learned some details about the accident. She'd been driving her car down a two-lane highway when a semi-truck crossed the center line and hit her head on. He also was intoxicated. She was completely justified in her anger; however, it still was destroying her life. One cannot be happy without forgiveness.

It's difficult for a chronic pain patient to move past fear in order to reach a loving state. There are many factors that create and reinforce fear, including wondering about the severity of the injury. Patients wonder, "How and when is it going to be resolved? How will I support myself? How can I be a good parent with this pain?" The anxiety and frustration becomes overwhelming. It's the antithesis of love and harmony. Becoming aware of how far you are from this mind set is an important step.

We discussed earlier that society has a vested interest in convincing you that you are less than whole. Chronic pain makes it worse, so you really don't feel whole. You think your life would be better without pain. I agree with that notion to a point; however, most of us probably didn't feel completely whole before the pain started and now it is accentuating the problem.

Flip the paradigm and instead of moving away from stress, move toward something good: practicing forgiveness, living your life based on love, and becoming whole. In doing these three things, you are choosing not to be a victim and living your life in peace.

## Awareness—Final Thoughts

Awareness is the first step in reprogramming your brain. It's important to spend as much time as possible doing active meditation, being fully aware of every stimulus coming into your brain. In other words, try to live your life in the first level of environmental awareness. When you wander into the second level of emotional awareness, just watch your emotions pass by and then pull yourself back into seeing, hearing, and feeling, as quickly as possible.

The third level of judgment/storytelling—for example, "the story"—is the most difficult for me. Once I am sucked into that level, it's hard for me to pull back. I will use active meditation but also have to use other methods, such as writing and visualization.

You need an outside perspective to become aware of ingrained patterns. It's impossible to see yourself clearly through your own eyes. Resources include psychologists, good friends, spouses, children, books, and seminars.

Becoming aware is much more interesting than constantly expressing and reinforcing your own views on life. Open yourself up to the world! The possibilities are infinite.

# CHAPTER 8

# Stimulating Your Brain to Change—Neuroplasticity

YOUR BRAIN IS IN A CONTINUAL AND DYNAMIC STATE of change depending on how much it is stimulated, or not stimulated. There is a name for this process—it's called *neuroplasticity,* which is defined as "the brain's capacity to adapt and change at any age." There is an incredible upside potential for us in the arena of neuroplasticity, as the nervous system has an almost unlimited capacity to evolve. The brain has about 86 billion neurons, all of which have multiple connections to each other. The number of connections is almost infinite.[1]

There are several ways that neuroplasticity occurs:

- Growth of new nerve cells (neurons).
- Shrinking of neurons from disuse.
- An increase or decrease in the number of connections per neuron.
- Creating or losing layers of myelin insulation. (This layer improves the speed of nerve conduction.)
- Substitution of an injured part of the brain from another functional area. (The new area takes on new capacities.)

Laboratory studies have revealed that that the brain actually shrinks in the presence of chronic pain.[2] It makes sense to me that if much of your brain is stuck in repetitive negative thought patterns, other areas—the ones connected to time with family and friends, enjoyable experiences, etc.—will atrophy. Additionally, adrenaline decreases the blood flow to your brain, which could be a factor.

A terrible consequence of brain atrophy is that you have less comprehension and ability to pull yourself out of the Abyss. But as discussed, chronic pain is a solvable problem; you just need help and tools. The fact you are reading this book is a promising sign. And brain shrinkage is not irreversible. Fortunately, the brain re-expands with resolution of the pain.

Brain changes occur quickly. With new fMRI technology, complex cross-wiring changes can be observed within a few weeks.[3] Additionally, it has been shown that when pain becomes chronic, brain activity shifts from the pain circuits to the emotional ones within six to twelve months. In other words, you are still experiencing the same pain but there is a different driver.[4]

## Your Programming

Your foundational programming happens during the initial ten to twelve years of life, when your brain absorbs everything in your environment. Negative behaviors and attitudes from your parents, friends, teachers and advertising seep into your consciousness. You also adopt labels, many of them negative, for almost every component of your life, including yourself. They evolve to become your "stories" and your identity. New and ongoing stimuli are interpreted through your labeling, which reinforces these stories.

You have a story about your chronic pain. I would venture to guess that it's not a positive one. Most of these stories are, in fact, quite dark; the only consistency I find is how well patients think they can hide their story from me and the pain psychologists with whom I collaborate.

Your story about chronic pain differs from your other stories in that it's associated with a physical sensation. This association makes the story particularly intense. The sensation of pain sparks negative thinking, which reminding you of your pain, which brings you back to your negative thoughts, and so on, creating new neurological pathways that are reinforced with repetition. Eventually, they become imbedded deeply enough to resist being broken or derailed. It has also been demonstrated that your pain becomes associated with more and more experiences and memories and therefore becomes more complex.[5]

Programming occurs for both emotional and physical pain, and the body's physiological response is similar. Since you cannot escape the sensory input generated by your thoughts, your body will be continuously bathed in stress chemicals and emotional pain may be the basis for chronic physical pain.

## Facilitating Neuroplasticity

There are two aspects to consider to successfully address the central nervous system component of pain: 1) the chemical environment and 2) the structure of the circuits. You must calm down the central nervous system to de-adrenalize it and stimulate the brain to rewire new circuits through neuroplasticity.

### *Decreasing the Stress Chemicals*

One of the core concepts of the DOC process is to simply calm down, which will decrease the levels of stress-induced hormones. It is the most direct way to alter your body's chemistry. Some of the methods include:

- Meditation is the practice of emptying your mind and keeping it that way for as long as possible. Intrusive thoughts are observed and let go. There are many types of meditation.

- Mindfulness involves placing your attention on sensory input and purposefully experiencing the details of your day.
- Active meditation is an abbreviated version of mindfulness.
- Cognitive behavioral therapy (CBT)—addresses distortions of thinking that keep you fired up by reinforcing your "stories."
- Medications can be a short-term adjunct to help calm you.
- Eating, unfortunately or fortunately, is relaxing and one of the reasons it is difficult to lose weight, especially if you are stressed.
- Expressive writing—separating "you" from your thoughts.
- Sleep, especially when you get a full night's sleep. The day's events are filed away and your brain refines your mental grid.
- Massage is a great way to relax and also have your brain focused on other sensations.

Pursue whichever of the above methods works best for you. Calming your nervous system is not the final solution, but it's almost impossible to move forward without this skill.

Animal studies in rats have shown that stress increases the conductivity of the peripheral nerves by 30 to 40 percent.[6] When threatened, living organisms will become more alert and hyper-vigilant, and the nervous system will change as a result of the stress chemicals. This causes you to feel more pain, which in turn adds to your stress. It's an endless cycle that can be broken only if you make the choice to use the tools for calming down.

### *Forming New Pathways*

We've established that your body's automatic response to any stress will always be one of survival. It happens instantaneously and it's powerful. Until you create an awareness of this unconscious reaction and also some space from it, you are not going to be able to alter it. There are three aspects to forming alternative neurological pathways:

- Awareness
- Separation
- Reprogramming

The various methods of stimulating neuroplasticity will be discussed in the context of these three aspects.

## Awareness

Awareness is the essence of living an engaged, rewarding, and enjoyable life. As you become more aware of every positive and negative detail of your reactions, you can choose to go in whatever direction you wish. It is remarkably freeing.

You also cannot solve a problem that you cannot see; that's why awareness is so important. There are many other benefits: consider that it's much more interesting to listen and learn rather than to always give your opinion.

For many people, becoming aware begins their healing process in a dramatic way. The filter of their "story" is removed and they see life in a completely different light. Everything and everyone appears different. It is something that happened to me in the Hoffman Process.

Since I was young, I've been upset about many global problems, ranging from world hunger to human trafficking. My list has been endless. Of course, I took on the problems in medicine the same way. I made a decision not to waste my energy complaining about them but to focus my frustrations on finding and developing solutions. It sounded pretty good to me but there was something missing that I could feel but did not see.

I participated in the Hoffman Process, as discussed in Chapter 4. The first stage of the process takes you through steps to understand the family patterns of behavior that have been imprinted in your brain by your parents that are now manifesting in your life. Until you understand these patterns, you will not be able to see yourself clearly. You are just playing out your mother or father or both in every automatic reaction you have to stress. Any time you are anxious or upset, you are in a pre-programmed pattern. Once you become aware, you have a choice whether to stay in that pattern or not.

About halfway through the week-long process, I became aware that focusing my anger on finding a solution for what I feel is too much spine surgery was turning me into a zealot. Being a zealot is based on angry energy, which triggers that same reaction in others. It's not effective in stimulating change and is not much fun. It was also wearing me down. Hoffman is about connecting you to your authentic self by clearing out these patterns, as opposed to fixing yourself. I became aware of my zealotry and was able to make an immediate switch to moving forward based on awareness, love, and true concern for those I come in contact with. It was a remarkable moment and my life has never been the same. The problem is that post-Hoffman, I do have a lot more energy and enthusiasm and I put too much on my plate.

There are an infinite number of ways to create awareness but you do have to make a conscious choice to become aware and open to change. There is no end to change. The good news is that it's interesting and your ego will melt away. The resistance seems to arise from the fact that change initially increases anxiety, which we all hate. Once you become comfortable with anxiety, you are free!

### Meditation and Mindfulness

Meditation has been used for centuries to separate the person from her thoughts and to train her not to react to them. Meditation allows us to experience a deep awareness of our environment as well as our reaction to it. By focusing on sensations and keeping your mind empty you can become both aware and calm. By "seeing" your automatic survival reactions, you now have a chance to resolve them or keep separating from them. Skilled meditators have great control over their nervous systems.

Although meditation is the classic awareness tool, it is difficult to learn and practice while in pain. It seems that a lot of people, including me, spend more time thinking about their pain while meditating, which is frustrating and reinforcing of the pain. For some, meditation is a practice that can be started later in the DOC process.

Mindfulness is the practice of fully experiencing what you are doing at the moment. Examples include tasting your food, listening to sounds, and feeling the breeze. An important part of this approach is also to keep perspective on your life while maintaining a sense of gratitude and humility.

Active meditation is my term for abbreviated mindfulness. As many times throughout the day as I can remember, I attend to any sensation for ten to fifteen seconds. It shifts me away from my reactive pathways, calms me down, and lets me instantly see the futility of getting worked up over something I cannot control. I use this tool hundreds of times during surgery. I focus on light touch and creating a wonderful performance. I want every move I make to be a beautiful move. It has not only transformed my surgical experience; it has also caused me to become more consistent in my performance.

Expressive writing accomplishes the first two steps of reprogramming: awareness and separation. I call it "mechanical meditation." Getting my thoughts on paper clarifies what's in my head and also separates me from them. It gives me the space to consider my reactions and substitute a more functional response. Verbalizing your thoughts aloud (in private) has a similar effect.

The effectiveness of expressive writing has been documented in over two hundred research papers. A 2005 paper[7] reviewed the benefits for both adolescents and adults, which included improvements in the following areas:

- Immune system function
- Lung and liver function
- Mood
- Blood pressure
- Psychological well-being
- Working memory
- Work attendance
- School and sports performance
- Grade-point average

Research has tended to focus on negative writing but it has been shown that positive writing is also effective. The debate is not if it works but about how and why it is so effective. It takes a while to become a skilled meditator, but simply putting pen to paper can be done with no practice; that's why I have patients immediately begin expressive writing. Nothing much really changes until the writing begins.

As mentioned earlier, in 1987, Dr. Daniel Wegner and others wrote the classic paper on thought suppression, nicknamed, "White Bears."[8] According to the paper, whatever you try not to think about, you will think about more. And when you try to think about something, you will think about it less. His term for this problem was the "ironic effect." He also wrote an essay, "The Seed of Our Own Undoing," pointing out that the more well-intentioned you were, the worse the problem. If you are well-intentioned, the greater likelihood that you will suppress dark thoughts; malevolent people don't even interpret many of these thoughts as negative. What happens is that a random neurological connection resulting in an unspeakable thought becomes a "parasite" in your brain. Every time you do battle with it you have given it more power and eventually it becomes a "demon"—except that it is not who you are. It is who you are *not* and it is an irrational circuit. Keeping these thoughts "out of mind" consumes a lot of life's energy. Wegner pointed out that expressive writing was probably the most appropriate tool to address this problem.[9]

Thought suppression is the antithesis of awareness. There is a growing body of evidence showing its damaging effects and it is considered to be the root cause of many illnesses and addictions.[10, 11]

*My Unawareness—and Its Consequences (OCD)*
I succeeded in suppressing my anxiety until I was in my thirties. I was a doer and plowed ahead regardless of adversity. Not succeeding was not an option. I always felt in control. Control is the logical and effective response to anxiety. However, it's also not conducive to rich and rewarding relationships.

I was raised in a difficult family situation full of anxiety and anger. It was the norm. All I knew is that sometime during my mid-teenage years, I decided I didn't like it, so I shut the door on my past on moved on. At the time, it seemed like a good idea and in retrospect, it was all I could have done. However, the psychological term for this is "dissociating." It represents an extreme form of mental suppression of anything negative and, indeed, I was quite successful in having a great and enjoyable life.

Eventually, dissociating had significant consequences. Also in the first year of my residency, I began to have intrusive thoughts. About ten years later, I suddenly began experiencing panic attacks and was forced to acknowledge anxiety as a personal problem. A panic attack is a set of symptoms that occur when your body releases adrenaline without a precipitating reason. I was driving across a bridge in Seattle about 10 o'clock at night after a long day. Suddenly my heart began to race, my chest was pounding, I broke out in a cold sweat, and I thought I was going to die. The attack occurred out of the blue. At that point I sought care and learned that, like the rest of the human race, I have anxiety.

My anxiety progressed into an obsessive-compulsive disorder (OCD). I never had any of the common outward manifestations of the disorder, such as hand washing or counting. Instead, I had what's called "internal OCD." With internal OCD, you have repetitive, intrusive thoughts that are answered by "counter-thoughts." The more I fought these thoughts, the more vivid they became. Needless to say, the process took up most of my emotional energy for fifteen miserable years.

## Separation

You are not your thoughts. Many philosophers have taught this concept for centuries. Thoughts are real but not your reality. I feel the reason that we give them so much attention is that our bodies chemically respond to every thought, whether it is positive or negative. We *feel* relaxed or agitated; we don't just think it. Cognitive scientists have long known that the mind and body respond to the environment as a unit.[12] There is no separation in the response unless you create it.

Separation is creating space between the stressor and your response. There are many ways to accomplish this. For many, just becoming aware of the neurological basis of physical and emotional pain instinctively allows them to pause enough to realize that their usual responses to the environment aren't working well and are often destructive.

Skilled meditators are able to separate from their distressing thoughts by visualizing them, watching them "pass through," and training themselves not to react to them. However, this is a challenging skill to learn and can be difficult to master while suffering from severe ongoing pain.

Expressive writing creates awareness and separation in one step. Your thoughts are now on paper and the separation is connected to you by vision and feel. Both are also part of the unconscious brain. It is simple, mechanical, and doable. That is why it's always the starting point of the DOC project. Until you can create some separation, you cannot engage in the DOC process, and the writing makes this happen.

The author David Burns's three-column technique[13] accomplishes separation as you categorize your thinking into one of the ten errors of thinking. As you write and classify the thoughts you can more clearly see the irrational nature of these universal cognitive distortions.

Thinking before you act or speak also creates a separation. It is common sense advice that we don't usually use. Considering the impact of your actions before you act is a powerful way to create separation between your thoughts and your actions. One of the reasons that anger is so deadly is that the opposite scenario kicks in. The blood supply to your brain decreases and since it is an intense survival reaction, you are acting quickly and with conviction of the rightness of your ways. Not surprisingly, there are usually negative consequences.

In an example of how this plays out, consider a situation where your seventeen-year-old son just let you know that his girlfriend is pregnant. I think most of us would experience an intense response and act on it quickly—but not constructively.

A better alternative would be to become aware of your negative thoughts and identify the actual stressor. This may seem obvious: "My son got his girlfriend pregnant. That's what's causing my stress." However, it's more complicated than that. By stressor, I'm referring to the specific aspect of the situation that's causing you to feel upset. Your son did not physically harm you or insult you. While he is your child, he *is* living his own life. And it shouldn't be a surprise that teenagers engage in sexual activity. It may directly affect you in that you'd feel obligated to provide physical and emotional support. However, you still have the choice of whether to do so or not.

So what's upsetting you? Perhaps it's that he violated your belief system; maybe you'd hammered away at him about the immorality of pre-marital sex, and you're upset he didn't take your belief to heart. Or he might have upset your image of the perfect family. For many cultures, however, this situation wouldn't be a problem. For most of human history people had children in their early teens and that is when you are the most apt to become pregnant and deliver a healthy baby. Many parents are excited to have a grandchild, whether or not there has been a wedding. The bottom line is that you are working from your *own* frame of reference.

It isn't a matter of being right or wrong, but rather realizing that if you're feeling stressed about a situation, it's critical to step back and look at it from a different perspective. As it becomes clear what part of the problem is the source of your stress, you will create the space you need to reprogram. You will also increase your chance of maintaining a healthy relationship with your son and helping him with his new responsibilities.

*Forgiveness*
Forgiveness is the ultimate strategy for achieving separation and creating the space you need between stressor and reaction. Why? Because in the act of forgiving, you let go of anger. When you're angry, you have greatly reduced awareness of your stressor and less control over your reactions. Anger keeps you mired in the past, and forgiveness is the only strategy that can really break you loose. Once you've forgiven whoever you're blaming for your unhappiness, you'll be able to see things more clearly and respond to situations more constructively.

Reprogramming
Awareness and separation begin the process of rewiring your brain by allowing you to see your programming. Once you have this level of

awareness, you can engage in reprogramming your nervous system via positive substitution, the final and necessary step in this sequence. The idea is to substitute negative thoughts and activities with more enjoyable thoughts and activities, creating new and more functional circuits.

There are an unlimited number of reprogramming methods, such as listening to music, re-engaging with friends and family, pursuing hobbies, and others. I will present some examples to illustrate the concept.

### Visualization

Visualization techniques have been used in the athletic and performing arts worlds for many years with numerous studies demonstrating the effectiveness of this method.

When you're in chronic pain, visualization can help you see a new life for yourself. Part of the chronic pain experience is feeling stuck, like your life will never change. But if you can picture a different existence—a time when you can move with greater ease and do more things—you can change your world. Visualizing a different life will displace your feelings of vulnerability and reprogram your brain in line with your hopes.

My son, Nick, was on the U.S. developmental ski team as a mogul skier. As I've mentioned, he's an excellent skier and has come close to making it all the way to the top. He and his best friend, Holt, have enhanced their performance skills by using both awareness and visualization in training. By using these techniques, they have not only elevated their performance, but have improved their ability to handle the inevitable failures that are inherent in any sport.

In March 2007, our family was watching the competition for the U.S. national championship in moguls. Nick had had a bad day and did not make the finals. Everyone, including Holt, was pretty upset. Nick had been talked into trying a trick he hadn't mastered, and he just didn't make it. Holt had a great run and qualified second. The top skier on the U.S. ski team had qualified third. The top twelve skiers out of a field of fifty get a second run and there are no carry-over of points from the first run.

The final run was winding down around 4 p.m. The sun was low and the light was flat. Flat light makes it much harder to see the shapes of the moguls. The top U.S. skier took his run and it was almost flawless. He scored a 27.2 out of a possible score of 30. Usually a score above 26.5 has a high chance of being the winning score. Holt was the next skier. We all were wishing him the best but just hoped that he would have a good run and possibly finish second or third. He came out, scored a 27.6, and won the U.S. championship. We were ecstatic and dumbfounded. It was an incredible run under any circumstances, but almost impossible to pull off under those conditions and that kind of pressure. At that point, I didn't really understand the visualization process and how it was different from positive thinking. So I spent the next day picking Holt's brain, asking how he was able to perform so well.

Here's what he told me. First of all, it's critical for the performer to acknowledge the anxiety associated with the upcoming performance. Holt was very anxious and knew that the score he had to beat was high. However, instead of suppressing his anxiety, he stuck with it and experienced it. He made a simple and quick choice: "I am not going to be controlled by any negative thoughts or emotions." He then turned his attention to active meditation. He felt the wind on his face and listened to the sound of his skis pushing against the snow. He felt himself breathe and just put himself onto the performance pathway he had visualized so many times. He didn't picture himself on the winner's podium, but rather focused on being present during the actual run mentally experiencing each move. The former is positive thinking, which would have distracted him from executing at his best. He had been practicing these techniques the whole season.

Holt said his past strategy would have been to suppress his negative emotions with thoughts like, "Don't worry about the other skier's score," "Don't be nervous," and "I can do it." The energy spent on trying to deny and cover up his real feelings would have taken away from the energy and focus he needed to perform. Instead, he chose an alternate neurological pathway that was the one he needed to maximize his performance.

The reprogramming that Holt did through visualization is a powerful method that is a little more advanced than writing exercises: with visualization, you experience the entire event in your head. It's the only program that's playing. It's important to go over each detail, from beginning to end.

Holt's method is validated by sports performance literature, which states that internal visualization is more effective than external visualization. With internal visualization, you actually *feel* as if you are performing the athletic feat, whereas with external visualization, you are merely watching yourself perform the event. You should be trying to feel the air, hear the crowd, and feel as much of your body moving as possible. The more senses you can experience in your mind, the better.

Visualization techniques can be applied in your life, not only in helping with your chronic pain but also in mundane day-to-day tasks.

*Play*

A few years ago as I was thinking about my own ongoing journey out of pain, I hit on the thought that, although anxiety, anger, and pain pathways are permanent, so are play pathways. It seemed to me that the problem was that they became buried by life, specifically by progressive anxiety. I made a decision that I was going cultivate a sense of play, regardless of the venue. After all, I enjoyed my work. I have always enjoyed my patients. The operation room became a performing arts theater. I viewed the hospital politics as opportunities and challenges. My life changed and I am having a great time despite my circumstances being the same. Enjoying my day is a learned skill that I continue to nurture daily.

Play can and will pull you upward out of the Abyss. It requires creativity that will light up an immense part of your brain. Aside from cultivating playfulness in your day-to-day life, you can learn a new skill or re-engage in something that you used to do, such as play an instrument, or play a sport. Believe it or not, those pathways are also permanent, even though you may not be connected to them or remember what they are like. They can be re-awakened. As your brain is engaged in this degree of complex, widespread, and stimulating activity, the pain pathways will quickly become uninteresting and eventually dormant.

### Gratitude: Changing Your Story

The burnout rate among physicians is over 50 percent and on the rise. It is a multi-factorial problem; but I think a contributing factor is the way we view life in medicine. I have a friend who is a general surgeon and a hard worker. He dislikes the politics of medicine and the emergence of so many rules and policies. I have to agree with him that this trend has not been helpful in improving the delivery or quality of care, and it borders on disruptive. He was telling me one day that, as soon as he takes his first step out of his car in the morning, he immediately begins to hate the hospital administration. He may have a legitimate gripe, but this mindset is certainly not helping him enjoy his day. An alternative would be to consider the opportunities he has to help people with their problems and provide relief. This is a privilege that he also appreciates.

What would his day be like if he consistently chose that way of thinking instead? He could express his contempt in the morning on a piece of paper, tear it up, and then go on to fully engage with his day.

One story that demonstrates the power of mindset is when my daughter, Jaz, was about thirteen and we were helping my wife host a tango party at her dance studio. Once a month she held an all-night milonga for about a hundred people. Jaz and I were not that happy to be there and she was already in a bad mood. I was about ready to give up trying to encourage her to cheer up when I had an idea. I said, "Look, I will give you twenty dollars if you can be happy for the next hour. You can't pretend and you have to be honest with me if you accomplish it." Much to my surprise, she not only took me up on it, but she had a great time the rest of the evening. She ended up connecting with a lot of friends who were glad to see her. Even now when she dips into a negative mood I will remind her about that evening.

Another example is a friend who was in dental school at the same time I was in medical school. We remained close after graduation. He set up his dental practice in a small town and was reasonably successful. However, he was not happy. He was too isolated, it was hard to find consistently good help, he wasn't living where he wanted to and the list of problems went on and on. About a year later, when I spent a weekend with him, he was a different person, energized and excited about building his practice and enjoying the community. But nothing else had changed. I asked him, "What happened?" He replied, "I decided to enjoy what I do." That was it. He continued to grow the practice to the point where he could, after which he sold it and moved back to his hometown.

## Stimulating Your Brain to Change—Neuroplasticity—Final Thoughts

One experiment that demonstrates the power of rewiring is one by the famous Russian researcher Ivan Pavlov. Pavlov showed how the brain could be trained, through repetition, to have certain reactions to specific stimuli. He is most known for his work in setting up an experiment where every interaction that a dog had with food would involve the sound of a bell. Eventually, just the bell sound would cause the dog to salivate, even without seeing or smelling food.

In one of his lesser-known experiments, he coupled the dog's feeding with an electric shock to one leg. With repetition, the dog would eventually seek the electric shock to obtain food and wouldn't react to the shock with a pain response. This phenomenon was "paw dependent" in that if the same shock was applied to its other leg, the dog would scream with pain.[14]

Ballet dancers place over a hundred pounds across the ball of one foot for hours and yet do not feel pain. In fact, they report deep emotional satisfaction.[15] Why is that? It is programming. What about football players and fighters? With controlled repetition the pain threshold can be markedly raised.

Conversely, with a disorder such as *reflex sympathetic dystrophy (RSD)*, the patient often cannot tolerate the touch of clothing. RSD is an imbalance of the sympathetic nervous system that results in extreme hypersensitivity to sensation. It is one of the most intense pain syndromes. Temporal mandibular joint syndrome (TMJ) is not too far behind. It is worsened as the sufferer continues to protect it.

I was taught in medical school that we are born with a finite number of neurons that we would gradually lose over our lifetimes, never to be replaced. I don't believe the word neuroplasticity even existed. Today we know that the capacity of the brain to dynamically respond to the environment is stunning. You have, and always have had, choices and responsibilities in the sculpting of your brain.

# SECTION 3:
# YOUR ROADMAP OUT OF PAIN

# CHAPTER 9

## Embarking on Your Journey

THERE ARE THREE PARTS TO THE DOC PROCESS, which is the self-directed program to define your own care: understanding chronic pain, addressing all the relevant variables, and taking charge of your own care.

While it may be tempting to turn your care over to a health care provider, the reality is that you know a lot more about your pain and how it may have evolved than anyone else. You can build on that knowledge by becoming aware of all the issues involved; this begins the healing process. Once you have direction and hope, your nervous system will begin to calm down, creating a more favorable chemical environment in your body.

### The Variables

The DOC process addresses six core areas, all of which have been shown in hundreds of research papers to significantly affect both surgical and non-surgical outcomes. They are:

- Education—awareness of the problem and solutions
- Sleep

- Medication
- Physical condition
- Stress
- Life outlook

The DOC process will be presented in four stages:

- Stage 1: Laying the Foundation
- Stage 2: Reactive to Creative–Forgiveness and Play
- Stage 3: Moving Forward
- Stage 4: Expanding Your Consciousness

### *Fighting a Forest Fire*

In my experience, many patients have a relentless drive to find the *one* answer that will resolve their pain. But there is no one answer. Many strategies are needed to resolve your pain and the choices will depend on your specific needs.

One useful analogy is that of fighting a forest fire. There are guidelines to creating a successful game plan; firefighters must assess the situation and conditions, figure out what methods they need to use, and then take advantage of the multiple resources at their disposal. Finally, there are protocols of engagement.

Local brigades extinguish most wildfires quickly with early detection. This is similar to health care, where early intervention is the one factor that consistently improves outcomes and also prevents a given situation from spinning out of control.[1]

If a fire is too large for the local brigade, a general call for help is sent out. The first fire chief to arrive on the scene is the one in charge; he or she sets up a base of operations and coordinates the effort. The main thrust of this effort is containing the fire and taking away its fuel. It requires multiple strategies, depending on factors such as the height of the flames, local terrain, and weather.

Now let's look at the parallels with chronic pain: with pain, *you* are the first fire chief on the scene; in other words, you are the one that must take charge. You are a unique individual and even if your doctor could spend hours assessing your situation, he or she couldn't know your life well enough to solve your problems.

When you're in pain, the fuel for the fire includes lack of sleep, adrenaline stimulated by anxiety and anger, inflammation, stiff tissues, lack of conditioning, high-dose narcotics, and dwelling on your pain. There are so many factors—it's not logical to think that there would be one solution for your pain, such as surgery.

Surgery is frequently considered the cure-all and the definitive solution for pain. But this is simply not the case. Without addressing the above factors, all of which adversely affect the perception of pain, surgical outcomes are poor more often than they are successful. In fact, with surgery, you can cause or exacerbate pain up to 40 percent of the time. The induction of chronic pain is seldom mentioned as a complication of surgery.[2]

In our current medical climate, most surgeons are not dealing with any of the pain variables that have been discussed in this book. A 2014 paper showed that surgeons addressed the known risk factors for poor outcomes only about 10 percent of the time.[3] I routinely see patients referred to me for surgery, who have not slept well for years, are experiencing severe anxiety, and are understandably angry. How well do you think an operation is going to work for those patients?

## Overview of the Process
### *Stage 1—Laying the Foundation*
My initial intention with patients is to slow everything down—especially

medical care—so they can learn about chronic pain and then begin to formulate a game plan. Stage 1 consists of these four steps:

1.  Begin doing the expressive writing exercises for five to fifteen minutes, twice a day. Write freely, preferably by hand, any positive or negative thoughts, paying no attention to grammar or legibility. When you're done, rip up the paper immediately; this will allow you to write with freedom. Expressing your thoughts out loud, in private, is also effective; but writing is the foundation and starting point of the DOC process. I want my patients to begin writing the night of their first appointment with me, even before they have done much reading. It is remarkably powerful, especially in light of its simplicity.

2.  Start doing active meditation exercises, drawing attention to your senses in the present moment. Practice this mindfulness activity five to fifteen seconds, as many times as you can throughout the day.

3.  Consistently get a good night's sleep. Refer to Chapter 14 for specific recommendations. Adequate sleep is one of the pillars of the DOC process; I won't proceed with any operative intervention in an elective case until a patient is sleeping well.

4.  Understand the neurophysiologic nature of chronic pain. If you have stuck with me this far into this book, you are well on your way.

### Stage 2—Forgiveness and Play

When the book *Forgive for Good* by Dr. Fred Luskin[4] became a core part of the DOC process a few years ago, more patients began to become free of pain. Forgiveness allows you to let go of the anger that tethers you to your past and prevents you from healing. The benefits of forgiveness are many; one is that it decreases your body's stress hormones. When patients practice forgiveness, I see their pain improve quickly. Dr. Luskin has taught me that forgiveness is a process that continues indefinitely. The first and most important person to forgive is yourself.

Play is a powerful reprogramming tool. Like pain pathways, play pathways are permanent, buried somewhere in your brain. Reconnecting with these circuits is the fastest way out of your pain. By "play" I am not referring to obsessive recreation; rather, it's about having fun and adapting a playful attitude to life. You can reawaken circuits from your past—activities you used to enjoy—or you can choose to approach your day-to-day tasks more playfully. You cannot truly relax and play if you are holding on to your anger. Remaining angry isn't much fun.

### Stage 3—Moving Forward

If your life has been disrupted—or destroyed—by pain, it's necessary to regroup. The DOC approach enables you to start this process, and usually people feel much better somewhere between Stage 1 and Stage 2. At this point, patients often quit using the DOC tools. This isn't a good idea, however. The key to sustained healing is to go through all four stages, which help you to pursue a full and productive life; it's the best way to keep your nervous system calm. Some practical ideas to stay on track include:

1. Create a vision for your life. You cannot travel anywhere without knowing where you want to go.
2. Address family issues. Anger destroys almost everything—especially your family. Rebuilding your family support system is important for your healing but also for your family's well-being.
3. Get organized. Your life has been focused on your pain and much of your life is in a state of disrepair. Getting organized is

a skill that you can learn from books, seminars, or the Internet.

4. Commit to a daily practice. Changing neurological pathways requires repetition. By committing to a daily plan that can be as short as five to ten minutes, you will continue to heal.

5. Think about the life you desire and connect with it. The further along you get with the DOC process, the more energy you will have to do this.

### Stage 4—Expanding Your Consciousness

The ultimate goal of the DOC process is to calm your nervous system and shift your brain onto a set of circuits that are more functional and enjoyable. Here are some suggestions:

1. Step into your new life with or without your pain. Perhaps the biggest paradox of this whole journey is that, if you move forward regardless of your pain, it's much more likely that your pain will disappear. Otherwise your pain will still be in control.

2. Embark on your inward journey. When you've disentangled yourself from the morass of anxiety and anger, you will be able to dive back through them and discover who you really are.

3. Fail well. Your pain pathways are permanent and life will keep coming at you. You may "fail" on a daily basis, with some days and weeks worse than others. It is important not to fight it, but to use your tools to learn from it and heal more quickly.

4. Go on a spiritual journey. Whatever form it takes, it's important to regain your sense of perspective and understand the importance of every minute of your human existence.

5. Give back. This step is the final manifestation of your healing journey. Being actively concerned about others is the ultimate shift of your consciousness to a bigger vision.

## The Paradoxes of Resolving Pain

The ultimate paradox of dealing with chronic mental or physical pain is that it becomes unresolvable by trying to resolve it. What do I mean by unresolvable? Often patients get stuck in the mindset of wanting to analyze and "fix" their pain so that it goes away and never returns. But you can never get rid of your pain circuits; they will always be there and can be triggered by a stressful situation at any moment. It happens to me fairly often. If you analyze your pain in order to remedy it, your attention will remain squarely on the pain!

This situation is problematic because the solution lies outside of our usual perception of how to problem solve. A normal sequence for dealing with a problem is to assess it, create a choice of solutions, and implement the best one. But with chronic pain the sequence is different. It goes like this: become aware, separate from the stressor, and move in a new direction.

Let's compare the two methods—the traditional model of picking the best solution versus the awareness-based model used in the DOC process—as they would play out in one scenario. Imagine that you were going to an important business interview. You'd think about what to wear and choose the appropriate attire. Then you'd get to the interview, see what others were wearing, and assess your appearance in comparison to them. If you thought you were under- or over-dressed, you might regret your choice of clothes and feel stuck, with no solution. After all, you can't go home and change. Your anxiety might rise, detracting from your performance.

In an alternate scenario, you get dressed, go to the interview, assess your appearance and see that you're over- or under-dressed. This time, however, you accept that what's done is done. Instead of worrying about it, you decide to relax, listen to and engage your potential boss, and enjoy the opportunity to have a shot at the position. Your performance is better than if you were letting your "appearance pathways" run the show.

Using the awareness/separation method takes practice—you need the tools to let go of things you cannot influence. But doing so allows you to place your mind exactly where it needs to be.

•••••

Keep in mind that any time spent trying to "fix" your negative pathways by eliminating them is counterproductive, because in paying more attention to them, you reinforce them. For instance, imagine that a traumatic event happened in your childhood and as an adult, you are fearful of similar situations. Although you might want to undo the event or get rid of your reaction of fear, it's impossible. The past is over and you can't change it or the links to it. Instead, you need to rewire your brain so that you're developing new, more functional and enjoyable pathways.

## Kelly's Story

Not long ago I had the privilege of talking to Kelly, the daughter of a friend, who was suffering from extreme chronic pain. Now in her mid-twenties, she has been struggling for years with crippling anxiety and multiple physical symptoms. She visited several physicians and tried every possible treatment without success. She was becoming despondent.

On the positive side, Kelly was a fast learner and incredibly open to new ideas. I was able to spend a few hours with her and explain the NPD treatment principles. As soon as she understood that she'd been spending most of her time trying to resolve unresolvable neurological problems, her eyes lit up. She understood that it was time to move on from the idea that there was only one possible resolution to her pain.

She started expressive writing, used active meditation, adopted an anti-inflammatory diet, and focused on getting more sleep. Within a few weeks she began to heal. A year later she was moving on with her life with minimal pain. I have been fascinated with how many people can blow out of their pain pathways relatively quickly, and how almost everyone succeeds with persistence. When people let go of unresolvable issues, they often experience a surge of energy.

## Flawed Strategies

There are several commonly used approaches to resolving pain, all of which are counterproductive. They include:

- Positive thinking
- Mind over matter, or sheer determination
- Talking it to death

### *Positive Thinking*

Earlier in the book we touched briefly on  positive thinking; the topic warrants further discussion, given the damage it can cause. Positive thinking has long been touted as one of the keys to a happy life. Unfortunately, this is a misconception; in fact, positive thinking was the habit that took me down. The path to becoming a complex spine surgeon is indescribably stressful, and surgeons aren't taught even the most basic stress management tools. So the only alternative seems to be positive thinking. It works for a while, but when it stops working, your anxiety takes over.

We discussed how humans have evolved around avoiding anxiety and consistently taking action to remain safe. Unfortunately, we have the habit of thinking troublesome thoughts and perceiving them as signifying danger, which causes the same chemical reaction as if there were real physical danger. For many, it seems the best way of dealing with these thoughts is to suppress them. Positive thinking is a form of suppression.[5]

Positive thinking occurs in the conscious part of the brain and has no chance of suppressing your body's powerful survival reaction. It is a gross mismatch. Although you may keep your mind in a positive place, your body's response to the negative input (your pain) will continue.

Positive thinking clouds awareness to the point where you cannot assess the true nature and extent of your problem. The only way to rewire your brain is to remain aware, create some space, and substitute healthy thoughts for unhealthy ones.

### Mind over Matter

The "mind over matter" approach creates the same problem as positive thinking. You cannot will yourself out of chronic pain; you will still be doing battle with monstrous circuits. You might as well be punching a wall or pushing a rock up a hill.

One patient who was especially determined to resolve her pain was the daughter of a friend, a woman in her early twenties who was suffering from chronic neck pain. Her energy and focus were admirable. She had done hours of research on every possible treatment. She was doing physical therapy, stretching, meditating, and getting acupuncture treatments. She hung a large flow chart on her wall that documented all of her treatments, as well as her pain. She found me because she was getting worse. To summarize a complicated conversation, I said, "The first thing you need to do is relax." This interaction is typical and frustrating to my patients. In this case, I was not answering her question about exactly which steps she needed to take to get better. Of course, I had her start by taking down the flow chart. She will eventually do well if she sticks with it, but the story is still evolving.

A Chinese finger trap is a good metaphor for trying to will yourself out of chronic pain. The finger trap is a device that orthopedic surgeons use to reduce fractures of your upper extremities. The patient is usually lying down with a cast holding the broken bones in alignment, and several fingers are placed into a device that encloses each finger in a nylon net. The idea is to suspend the arm and create a distracting force across the fracture to reduce it. As more weight is placed on the arm or you try to pull out of it, the nylon netting around the fingers tightens and becomes stronger. If this apparatus is placed properly, it's impossible to break out of it.

Treating chronic pain is similar. The harder you try to escape or push through the pain, the more you will become enmeshed in it. Conversely, if you use the tools to calm your nervous system, you will have started the healing process. Relaxing tension is the first step in taking off the Chinese finger trap.

### *Talking It to Death*

If you're in chronic pain, it may be tempting to discuss your pain with anyone who will listen. But this actually prevents healing. Why? 1) It reinforces pain pathways; and 2) the time you spend complaining takes away from time spent on enjoyable and creative experiences.

Several papers have documented that belonging to a pain support group is a predictor of a poor prognosis for healing.[6] One explanation is that the format might encourage interaction in a way that reinforces each other's suffering. Monitoring your pain with a pain diary has also been shown to factor into a poor prognosis for chronic pain. This is a common practice that is suggested by physicians, and yet the data indicate that it's not helpful.[7]

Complaining also drives others away; social isolation is common among those in chronic pain. Unfortunately, this isolation gives you more time to spend on your pain pathways. We have demonstrated that people who are socially isolated and people in chronic pain activate the same parts of their brains. Being alone is painful.

The other problem with complaining is that the people you do connect with are also suffering; this is your common bond. But relating to people by complaining is not a great way to create rich and fulfilling relationships.

Do you enjoy being around negativity? How do you think others feel being around you when you're in a bad mood? If these are the people you *do* really connect with, then you need to step back and take a look at who you are.

I realized the extent to which people in pain complain when I ran a pain workshop at the Omega Institute in Rhinebeck, New York. There was initially a lot of conversation around the participants' pain and medical care, but then we instituted three ground rules: 1) no sharing details of your pain; 2) no discussion of medical care; and 3) no complaining—period. Most participants were thrown off by not being able to discuss their pain but came to realize how important it was in contributing to their healing.

Much of each workshop was focused on play and sharing. In addition to being a tap dancer, my wife Babs is a movement expert. She led the play segments. As people let go of control and relaxed during her part of the week's sessions, their pain diminished. We were shocked at how quickly and completely chronic pain could disappear. If you pay attention to your pain day in and day out, you *can't* rewire. How much time do you spend thinking (obsessing) about your pain? How aware are you of others' needs? What percent of your conversations are spent discussing some aspect of your suffering? Do you really enjoy discussing your pain? Don't you become tired of it? How can you enjoy your life when you are continually upset?

## Embarking on Your Journey—Final Thoughts

Implement Stage 1 of the DOC program before you move on. It's the foundation of the rest of your journey. Without understanding pain, getting adequate sleep, doing expressive writing and active meditation, you cannot move forward.

The rest of the phases are interrelated. I challenge my patients to think creatively and to think large. Many of us have become so used to having a survival mindset that we've accepted it as our norm. What happened to the dreams you had in high school? Do the words peace, love, and joy resonate with you? What about play?

When people get stuck it's usually because they have quit expressive writing. Invariably, I am told about some family crisis or work situation that didn't allow them to write. Really? It takes five to ten minutes once or twice a day. The more intense your stress, the more important it is to practice the tools you've learned.

The other roadblock is forgiveness. People do not want to let go and forgive, but they are the ones who are suffering. Why would you want to do that, and how long do you want to do it for? The problem is that the victim role is so powerful that it is extremely difficult to give it up.

Often people will get past their anger, feel dramatically better, and then quit before Stages 3 and 4. I understand how this can happen, but the last two stages are where you get the tools for building a life that you can only imagine. It is the best part.

# CHAPTER 10

# Stage 1—Laying the Foundation

THE GOAL OF THIS CHAPTER IS TO HELP YOU BECOME AWARE of your situation, learn the basic tools of the DOC process, and prepare yourself for the rest of the journey. The DOC approach is intended to be simple, so that patients can easily internalize the core concepts. Too many treatments are complex and distracting. This first stage, laying the foundation, consists of five steps, all of which are considered in the context of awareness, separation from the stressor, and reprogramming your brain.

Here is an overview of the five steps:

**Step 1**: Learn About What's Affecting Your Pain (Awareness)
- Confirm your diagnosis
- List how many NPD symptoms you are experiencing.
- List the factors affecting your pain
  - Sleep
  - Stress
  - Medications
  - Physical conditioning
  - Life outlook

**Step 2:** Begin expressive writing (awareness and separation)

**Step 3:** Practice active meditation (reprogramming)

**Step 4:** Don't share your pain (reprogramming)

**Step 5:** Sleep (reprogramming)

## Step 1: Learn About What's Affecting Your Pain (Awareness)

You have spent a lot of time learning about chronic pain in this book. Now apply this knowledge to your situation.

### *Confirm Your Diagnosis*

It's crucial to understand your diagnosis even if it requires several doctor visits. Your problem will either be structural, non-structural, NPD, or a combination. If the source of your pain cannot be identified, that's good news; it means that your problem is more resolvable.

Unfortunately, it's rare for physicians to agree on the nature of one patient's problem, and the diagnosis of NPD is not yet part of mainstream medicine. Once it's been confirmed that you don't have a serious structural problem, move on.

### *NPD and You*

Even though I list NPD as a separate diagnosis, the truth is that you have NPD, regardless of any other structural or non-structural diagnoses. Everyone has at least three or four symptoms, whether or not they have pain. How many NPD symptoms do you have? Identify yours from the list of symptoms presented in Chapter 1, and compile your own list. By understanding the nature of NPD with its multiple symptoms, you can treat the root cause of a triggered and over-adrenalized nervous system. You won't have to treat each symptom as a separate problem. Keep this list.

To calm your nervous system, you must first identify the "triggers" to your past traumas. If a situation resembles a past traumatic event, then your whole body may unconsciously overreact to it. The trigger can be minimal, such as a voice or physical attribute that is similar to a person who may have abused you. This book is not intended to explore the origins of your triggers, although at some point in your journey this may become an important avenue to pursue. This triggering is the essence of PTSD, which is considered an NPD symptom.

Keep in mind that there is an important difference between becoming aware of a trigger and analyzing it. Spending time defusing the trigger won't work. However, knowing the trigger exists will help you understand your strong reaction to it.

### Other Factors

What are the other variables that are affecting your pain?

- Sleep
  - How many hours a night are you sleeping?
  - Is it restful or interrupted?
  - Are you tired the next day?
- Stress
  - Anxiety
    - How anxious are you?
      - Rank it on a scale from one to ten.
    - List ten situations that make you nervous.
  - Anger
    - What are you upset or frustrated about? Make a list of things that upset you.
  - Circumstances
    - It has been well-documented in multiple research studies that stress causes disease. Make an exhaustive

list of any stresses you have been struggling with in the last twelve months, including both positive and negative events. A famous study done in 1964 created a list of 43 stressors and quantified them.[1] Many of them are positive experiences, such as a new child, marriage, promotion, etc. Stress is stress.

- Medications
  - Make a list of prescription and over-the-counter medications and categorize them according to the reasons they have been prescribed for you.
    · Pain control
    · Decreasing anxiety
    · Improving sleep
    · Decreasing nerve pain
    · Medical problems
    · Other

## Step 2: Begin Expressive Writing (Awareness and Separation)

The first action I have my patients take is to start expressive writing. They write down their thoughts and then immediately destroy the paper. That allows them to write with freedom. Other suggestions include:

- Write either positive or negative thoughts or feelings.
- Write down specific thoughts and emotions exactly as they come to you.
- Just get your pen onto paper. Your writing doesn't have to be legible or logical. Scribbling or symbols will work.
- Write once or twice a day for fifteen to thirty minutes per session.
- If you initially find it too disturbing, stop or limit it. If you can't

get past this exercise, seek support and guidance from a mental health professional.

- Make it a lifetime practice. Eventually, just a few minutes a day will help you maintain your sense of well-being.
- Handwrite if possible. Handwriting is a complex task that converts thoughts into a motor function. Large regions of the brain are activated when you write by hand.[2]

You can also use the auditory route. Saying thoughts allows them to travel to your brain through a different set of circuits. David Burns, in his book *Feeling Good*, suggests an exercise where you stand in front of a mirror and talk to yourself using the self-critical voices in your head. You would never talk to another human being that way.[3]

Consider the writing as something you do automatically every day, like brushing your teeth. It's usually part of my daily routine but sometimes I drop off. During these periods, I predictably re-experience some NPD symptoms within a couple of weeks. My sleep quality drops, I am more reactive, my scalp itches, my feet burn, and two small skin rashes develop on both of my wrists. My wife will ask me, "Honey, have you been doing your writing?"

Over two hundred papers[4] have shown the power that writing has on the nervous system. Much of the research has focused on writing about negative thoughts or past traumas. The original paper in 1986[5] asked volunteers to write in detail about the most traumatic events of their life for twenty minutes a day for four consecutive days, and then compared them to a group who was just asked to write about their day. They were evaluated four months later, and the results were profound: the writing had a remarkably positive effect on both mental and physical health. They did note an initial dip in mood and sense of well-being with the group that wrote about trauma, but there were no major problems.

Historically, research about expressive writing has been focused on writing down negative thoughts or about prior traumas. More recent papers have shown that positive writing is as effective.[6] Somehow, expressing thoughts and feelings on paper changes the brain. The debate about the writing is not *if* it works but how and why it works.

Keep in mind that focusing on negatives without the guidance of a mental health professional may be too much for a given patient. There has been no major fallout from the writing, but there is no reason to dive deeply into negatives if positive writing works. Free writing of current thoughts and feelings is easier than dredging up the past.

Also remember that negative thoughts will surface on their own, with or without negative writing. You may feel like they are "issues," but they are just thoughts. Analyzing them strengthens them; writing them down helps you separate from them. The pain psychologist I work with has noticed that patients are better able to make progress when they write.

Here are some suggestions about what *not* to do when writing:

- Don't journal or keep these writings; it's counterproductive. I feel it represents the need to control these thoughts. Remember this is a separating and letting-go process and not a problem-solving one. Journaling is fine, but it is a different endeavor that does not accomplish the needed separation.
- Don't keep a notepad to write throughout the day. Patients sometimes view writing as a way to capture and fix their thoughts, but since there are trillions of thoughts in your brain, this isn't going to work.

### *Unhooking from the Train*
Picture yourself as the engine of a long, loaded freight train. You can pull

a tremendous amount of weight. It's similar to how we drag our past into the current day.

Expressive writing disconnects you from the past immediately. When I write, I become aware of my thoughts. The space created between the thoughts on paper and me is the separation process. It is as if I unhooked the first car from the engine. There is no rule of life that says I have to stay connected to that huge load. And I still have the same power of an engine that is now pulling *nothing*. The creative energy that becomes available is almost limitless. The constraints on creativity then become time and physical capacity—not anxiety.

### *The Three-Column Writing Technique*

*Feeling Good* is the book that initiated my journey out of the Abyss, and I will be forever grateful that I ran across it during such a critical period. David Burns said to write, so I began to write—a lot. I did not realize the importance of writing until much later.

In 1997 I began using the book clinically, as Burns pointed out that the exercises in it had been effective for anxiety and depression over 80 percent of the time. It was also much faster than trying to see a pain psychologist. For many years, *Feeling Good* was the mental health component of the DOC process. It was clear that the patients who did well were writing.

The first third of *Feeling Good* describes cognitive behavioral therapy. One of the tools is the "three-column" technique, which represents the three phases of reprogramming: 1) awareness, 2) separation, and 3) creation of a new pathway.
The three columns are:

| *Negative thought* | *Error in thinking* | *Rational thought* |
| --- | --- | --- |

By writing your negative thoughts in the first column, you are increasing your awareness of the problem.

An error in thinking could be any number of things, including "should thinking," "labeling," "mind reading," "catastrophizing," etc. Categorizing your error initiates the separation process. You are separating from your initial reaction. You then have a choice to either continue that line of thinking or to restructure your thoughts. In the third column, the more rational follow-up thought is written down, creating a new neurologic pathway.

Here's an example of the three-column technique in action. It's common for spouses to have different views on punctuality. You might always be on time while your spouse is habitually late. In this scenario, you'd likely have a similar set of thoughts every time he was late, such as, "My time isn't being respected" or "He's always late. He's an inconsiderate person."

If your spouse was late to meet you for an event one night and you were still stewing about it afterward, here's one way to process the situation. When you get home, take out a piece of paper, create three columns, and then fill them in:

| Negative thought | Error in thinking | Rational Thought |
|---|---|---|
| Inconsiderate | Labeling | I don't know why he was late. We'll discuss it later. |

You may have the same or similar thoughts the next time the lateness occurs, but by writing repeatedly, their frequency and intensity will diminish.

Another scenario would be your son flunking a test at school. Your first response might be, "He's lazy and stupid." Using the three-column technique, you'd write those thoughts down in the first column. In the second column you'd note that your thoughts were "labeling," "catastrophizing," and "overgeneralizing." In the third column you might write,

"My son just flunked a test. I wonder why? Is he being bullied at school? Could he be depressed? I need to try to find out what's going on."

Note that what you've done is different from positive thinking. With positive thinking, you would have written, "He isn't lazy. He's my son and I love him," and that might be it. Except, without writing a more specific rational response, your thoughts might start to spin around. By the time you actually talked to him, you might not be in a great frame of mind.

By writing about the situation, you are separating from your thoughts via touch and feel, and forming new pathways. I have observed very few patients who could bypass this step and become pain free.

## Step 3: Practice Active Meditation (Reprogramming)

Free writing creates awareness and separation. The third part of the sequence, reprogramming, can be accomplished in thousands of ways such as spending time with friends and loved ones, pursuing a hobby, listening to music, playing sports, and more. However, there is one core method that I feel is the starting point. I call it "active meditation" and it's a variation of mindfulness. Active meditation consists of simply placing your attention on sensations. Any one will do—taste, feel, sound, pressure, etc. There are three steps and it just takes five to ten seconds per time.[7]

- Relax: I often begin by relaxing my shoulders; you can use any body part. Or I take a deep breath.
- Let yourself stabilize: feel the body part you relaxed for a few seconds before going to Step 3.
- Focus on one sensation: taste, feel, sound, pressure, etc. Feel the vividness of the sensation increase.

Active meditation accomplishes several things. As you relax, your body secretes less adrenaline. By placing your attention on a sensation, your nervous system shifts off the pain pathways. With practice, it will become more automatic. Eventually, as you use the pain pathways less, they will become weaker and the other pathways will become stronger.

Active meditation is quick and allows you to connect with the present moment in the midst of chaos. Although free writing is best done a few times a day, I practice active meditation as often as I think of it. It has become more habitual with practice, and I succeed maybe twenty to thirty times a day.

### *Traditional Meditation and Mindfulness*

Traditional meditation practice is a tool that accomplishes all three steps. You become aware of your thoughts as you try to quiet your mind and train yourself not to react to them. Then you reconnect to the present moment, using whatever method you are the most comfortable with. It can be a great way to begin or end your day. There are many practices and you can find one that you relate to. Skilled meditators have an extraordinary capacity to relax and connect. I recommended meditation as my main tool for a couple of years but found out that is difficult to quiet your mind when you are experiencing pain.

When you fully experience every aspect of the activity you are involved in at the moment, you are using mindfulness—living your life in a purposeful and connected manner. Connecting with physical sensations is a significant aspect of this practice. Because it takes less time, I prefer active meditation, my abbreviated version of mindfulness. I am a strong proponent of mindfulness-based living as a way of physically connecting to your reality.

## Step 4: Don't Share Your Pain (Reprogramming)

Your brain will develop wherever you place your attention. Complaining will keep you stuck on unpleasant circuits. The longer you're stuck, the stronger the circuits become, and eventually they will bury you. I was one of those people who could and would complain about almost anything in detail, which included my mental and physical pain. It seemed incredibly important to me and I couldn't figure out why others were so uninterested. It was only after I began to heal that I could see how deadly it was to be constantly unhappy.

This step seems simple—but it's not. Start noticing how often you complain, and then just stop. Initially, you will fail frequently and also be at a loss for words. You will have to make a deliberate effort to read the newspaper, watch an interesting movie, read a good book, volunteer—anything to wake your brain back up. Almost everything is more interesting than your pain. Write down the complaints you would normally share with your friends and tear them up. Not sharing your pain is one of the more powerful tools for moving on.

## Step 5: Sleep (Reprogramming)

Sleep is the number one priority in the rehabilitation process. The only reason I put nervous system issues ahead of sleep in this chapter is that the calming tools will also help you sleep. None of the DOC principles will be effective if you are not getting seven or eight hours of restful sleep per night. Not one major decision regarding your spine care, especially surgery, should be made until you feel rested during the day.

Approach your sleep issues step by step. These are discussed in detail in Chapter 14.

The medical profession does not systematically assess or treat insomnia. You will have to make it your responsibility to get adequate sleep. There are many resources; and, even in the presence of pain, you can sleep.

## Stage 1—Laying the Foundation—Final Thoughts

You have come a long way on your journey out of pain. Many people feel so good using the methods in this stage that they quit. But finishing Stage

1 is just the starting point. You have built a foundation and are possibly out of the Abyss. You haven't even come close, however, to tapping your potential for stimulating your brain to rewire.

Stage 1 Suggested Reading

- *Feeling Good* by David Burns, M.D.: Read at least the first one-third of the book, to learn the three-column writing technique.
- *The Talent Code* by Dan Coyle

# CHAPTER 11

# Stage 2—Forgiveness and Play

BOTH HARD WORK AND CREATIVITY ARE IMPORTANT for devising new ideas and implementing them, both personally and in the business world. New ideas stimulate us and help us to thrive. One thing that stands in the way of this activity is anger. In fact, it's almost impossible to be creative if you're angry; it could be argued that anger is the antithesis of creativity. How so? When you're angry and focused on survival, adrenaline shuts down the blood supply to your brain. I feel that anger is temporary insanity.

## Reactive vs. Creative

ReaCtive

Creative

The difference between these two words—and these two concepts—is that in the word "creative," the "C" (which can mean see) is at the beginning. In "reactive," the "C" (see) is buried in the middle of the word.

It's impossible to be creative when you are in a reactive mode. Whenever you are anxious, or worse, angry, you are in a patterned, conditioned, automatic reaction. We all know certain phrases, behaviors, situations, and people that will elicit a fairly predictable and rapid reaction in us. We react before we have absorbed or comprehended the full scope of the situation.

The first step in effective problem solving is seeing all aspects of a given problem and then choosing how to respond. To be creative, you must first C/see.

Unfortunately, these programmed reactions become stronger with age and repetition. "You can't teach an old dog new tricks" is accurate to a certain extent. But it's not that the dog cannot be taught; it's that it must be open to being taught.

It is my opinion that our increased life span is one of the reasons our society is so angry and reactive. One of the greatest accomplishments of the twentieth century is a dramatic increase in life span. Much of it has been attributed to addressing communicable diseases through public health measures, such as clean water. Cardiac advances and antibiotics are major contributing factors, too.[1] Many think that increased stress is what causes us to be angry, but I disagree; human existence has always been challenging. It's just that now we have many more years of our negative circuits being reinforced. It's an unfortunate progression, especially considering how much better our physical living conditions are now, compared even just a hundred years ago.

Our current societal and political rhetoric is becoming harsher, as is our reactions to it. Instead of experiencing increasing wonderment and curiosity about all of our modern opportunities, many of us are becoming increasingly rigid and cynical.

A step each of us can take is to become aware of our own reactivity. The methods to disrupt the compulsive links of conditioned behavior are easily available, but they are not widely adopted. After first "C"-ing" both your global and day-to-day reactions, you will have the power to create choices that will energize your life. The "C" must be first.

## Steps to Reconnecting with Your Creativity

Here are six suggested steps to help you break away from your automatic reactive survival patterns.

### AWARENESS

Step 1: *Understand the impact of anger on your life*
Step 2: *Acknowledge your disguises*

### SEPARATION

Step 3: *Admit your victimhood*
Step 4: *Choose not to be a victim*
Step 5: *Forgive*

### REPROGRAMMING

Step 6: *Play*

### *Awareness*

Step 1: Understand the Impact of Anger on Your Life

As I said before, remaining angry causes increased pain and disability as well as a decrease in the quality of your life.[2] This is particularly true if you continue to blame others or situations for your problems. Why remain upset about a distant event or at a given person? How does hanging on to negativity help you enjoy your day?

Years ago, I was caring for a patient who'd undergone a successful disc excision that resulted in complete relief from her leg pain. But even though the surgery came out well, she still had a lot of vocational issues to deal with and was appropriately angry. She initially didn't see or acknowledge her anger, so several weeks after the surgery I finally convinced her to begin writing. She pursued it with a vengeance and even consented to see the pain psychologist I work with. She seemed to be doing well with both the stress-related issues and her spine, but then it all came to a halt. When I asked her how the writing was going about three months after surgery she replied, "I stopped. First, I realized that I was an angry person. Then, as I kept writing, I started to feel depressed. I'd rather be angry than depressed." I then had a very circular conversation with her for about twenty minutes before I finally gave up. I don't know what happened to her after that.

It was during this interaction that I realized how strong anger was in both covering up and reinforcing anxiety. While you are in the midst of feeling angry, you feel very little, if any, anxiety. I also feel that anxiety drives depression. In the short term my patient did feel more anxiety and depression. However, in the long-term she will have missed the opportunity to connect with herself and with the potential of living a better life.

## Step 2: Acknowledge Your Disguises

None of us likes the idea that we might be acting like a victim. We don't even like the word, and there are an infinite number of ways to disguise it, which were presented in Chapter 5. One of the problems with anger is that you feel so justified in your rightness that you cannot conceive of anyone disagreeing with you.

My go-to disguise is, "I'm frustrated." I did not realize for many years that frustration and anger were essentially the same thing. My list of disguises would truly fill a thick book, as this may be my most highly evolved life skill.

Write down the disguises you may be using. This exercise will provide you with better awareness of who you are. Save the list.

## *Separation*
### Step 3: Admit Your Victimhood
Use the following sequence to get in touch with your victim role:

- Ask yourself, "What person or circumstance is upsetting me?" Be specific.
- Acknowledge that you are blaming that person or situation for making you angry.
- Write or speak out loud to yourself, "I blame [so-and-so or such-and-such] for making me upset."
- Understand that you are now in the victim role, a universal feeling.
- Write or speak, "I am allowing myself to be a victim of [so-and-so or such-and-such]."

Clearly differentiate whether you are: 1) being truly victimized or 2) basing your victimization on a perception that comes from a "story" in your mind. Note how much more difficult it is to process the anger if you've been truly victimized.

Obviously, your chronic pain will be high on the list of circumstances that are making you feel like a victim. However, don't let this get in the way of identifying the multitude of other ways you might be playing that role. Any time you're frustrated or angry, you're in victim mode. Whenever you feel angry, instead of blaming someone (or something), take full responsibility. Learn to do the "admit your victimhood" exercise regularly.

For years I didn't recognize my anger. With my expertise in suppressing emotions, I fancied myself a very calm, cool, and collected person. In fact, one of my opening lines to my future wife in 2001 was that I was "one of the few people I knew who had really dealt with his anger issues." If either of us could have known what lay ahead. Things changed when my personal circumstances got so bad that I was forced to come face to face with my underlying rage—I couldn't escape the fact that it was one of my core patterns. I realized that while I'd dealt with my anxiety, anger was still a major factor in my life.

When I hit my core anger, it was like an oil gusher. It didn't feel good or cathartic in the least. It felt dirty, noxious, and despicable. However, it was only by becoming aware of it that my life could change. Within six months of confronting my anger (not by choice and not well) my thirteen-year battle with anxiety-driven burnout thankfully came to an end. I still frequently fall back into the victim role, but now I have the tools to quickly come out of it. It has been sobering to realize how much of my life I spent in that mindset. Now I feel much freer.

It's not uncommon for people to deny their anger issues. I often have patients who insist that life is great outside of their chronic pain, but anger keeps emerging in comments like, "The doctor did the wrong operation," or "How could I have had so many operations that didn't work?" The emotional tension is clear to me, but they can't see it. The elephant in the room is that their chronic pain is not compartmentalized; it resonates throughout their lives as a disability accompanied by anxiety, anger, and general unhappiness.

An example of this was a retiree who had been suffering from pain for over five years. It encompassed about half his body. He insisted he was happy and that he had nothing negative to write about. I have to admit that I get a little triggered when I hear that from one of my patients, because that was the pattern that took me down. I sat back in my chair, which is now my usual response, and asked him, Are you happy with your pain? He gave the predictable answer, "Of course not!" I couldn't resist pointing out that he now had something to write about.

Anger associated with chronic pain is real victimhood. That's why it's difficult to let it go. But it's crucial to acknowledge it—it's the only way to move forward with your recovery.

I confess that admitting to my victim status has been the most challenging part of my own journey. I went through a phase where I thought that I'd learned enough about being a victim and that I was above it. I considered myself enlightened. I was completely unaware and it was a challenging phase of my life.

## Step 4: Choose Not to Be a Victim

Once you get a clear sense of the depth of your anger and victimhood, make a simple decision not to be a victim anymore.

- Write down, "I choose not to be a victim." Date it and put it where you'll see it every day. Remember that:
  - It's an intellectual choice that needs to be accompanied by reprogramming tools in order to be effective. Victimhood is so powerful that you will never wake up one morning and feel like, "I don't want to be a victim anymore." You just have to make a mental choice.
  - You will repeatedly fail, and that's okay. Don't stop your efforts.
  - Commit to being honest with yourself.
- "Do" vs. "Try" (Hoffman Process concept)
  - "I will try" is the ultimate victim phrase. Write "try" on a piece of paper, cross it out, and hang it on your refrigerator.
  - Write "Do" on another piece of paper and hang it on your bathroom mirror.

*My Decision to Move On*

My history of abuse had a powerful effect on my life, and by 2001, I was in a terrible emotional state. I could barely make it through the day. Although I remained a technically excellent surgeon, I was miserable. I was in severe burnout and had pursued every possible avenue of help with a vengeance, but nothing seemed to work. In fact, I was getting progressively worse.

A life-changing moment for me occurred in May 2002. I was outside with my future wife and daughter, washing their car on a beautiful Mother's Day. I had every reason to feel happy. But instead of being happy, I was in mental agony, enveloped in crippling anxiety. This juxtaposition of the lovely day and my misery made no sense. I started thinking about how tired I was of all my internal unrest. Suddenly, I realized how I'd placed myself in the victim role. It hit me like a lightning bolt. That moment led me to a deep decision, one that would eventually pull me out of my despair: I would stop playing the victim. The sequence of events that brought me to that decision was complex, but the decision itself was simple. Within six weeks, my anger began to abate. Three months later, I'd made major changes in my life.

It took another year before I really pulled out of my tailspin, but my life took a crucial turn that weekend. One of my realizations was that I'd been on an endless pilgrimage to find the one solution that would relieve my suffering. I'd been searching for an outside source to solve my problems, continually looking to be fixed or find a way to fix myself, for good. That day, I realized that there was not one single solution that would fix me. Instead, I needed to adopt a multifaceted approach in an ongoing process. There would be no endpoint.

Then I returned to David Burns's book, *Feeling Good*.[3] At that point I wasn't aware of how to develop alternative neurological pathways—all I knew was that the book's exercises worked for me. Plus, I noted that the author said the book's cognitive restructuring was effective in relieving anxiety 85 percent of the time. I recommitted to Burns's writing and repetition techniques.

Years after I started the *Feeling Good* exercises, the Hoffman Process added several dimensions regarding the role anger played in my life.

## Step 5: Forgive

Forgiveness is an individual, personal process. Many books have been written on the subject over the centuries, but the book that's been the most effective for my patients and me is *Forgive for Good* by Dr. Fred Luskin.[4] In fact, it was a patient who first told me about it. Dr. Luskin, director of the Stanford University Forgiveness Project, has conducted four major research projects on this topic. In his book, he discusses the nature of true forgiveness and provides steps for achieving it. When this book became part of the DOC project, my patients began to experience a remarkable decrease in their pain. When patients get stuck, it is generally anger that is holding them back.

Somewhere in the midst of working through deep anger issues, a process that, by necessity, includes acceptance and forgiveness, chronic pain often diminishes or even disappears. Conversely, if you think about it in terms of circuits and connections, it's essentially impossible to decrease your pain without truly letting go of your legitimate anger. It's not a psychological issue; it's that the anger and pain circuits are intertwined.[5] Pain elicits anger and frustration. When other circumstances upset you, those circuits then fire up your pain pathways. One of the first things my patients notice after they understand this link is that stress really does increase their level of pain and, of course, pain increases their stress.

### Forgiveness Strategies

One important point Dr. Luskin makes about forgiveness is that it's a process, and deep emotions can be triggered throughout your life regardless of how much you think you have forgiven someone. The process involves the use of multiple tools that are beyond the scope of this book. I am going to list some of them here so you can get a glimpse of the range of possibilities.

The first thing Dr. Luskin explains is that forgiveness is only for you; it has nothing to do with the perpetrator. And it has to be real, deep forgiveness. Intellectually forgiving someone or something in your past has a positive effect, but it only scratches the surface compared to really digging in, feeling, and creating alternate, forgiving neurologic pathways. You do not have to like the person who harmed you. But you also do not have to mentally drag that person along with you for the rest of your life.

Some other of Dr. Luskin's suggestions:

- "Change the channel." You can choose the way you view a person or situation.
- Learn to view the world through your enemy's eyes.
- Understand that the person who angered you is not the problem. He or she triggered a pathway in you and your anger is your problem. Anthony de Mello, in his book, *The Way to Love*, takes it a step further by stating that it's important to learn to mentally thank the person who angered you, as he or she has provided you with insight into who you are.
- It is critical to take 100 percent responsibility for your anger, period.
- If you have complained about a situation more than three times to others, you have developed a "grievance story" where you are the victim. Get over it and move on.
- Train yourself to co-exist with anger. Instead of reacting, stay calm. Dr. Luskin taught me a meditation that involves lying on the floor and visualizing a difficult person or situation. I am supposed to remain calm and relaxed while holding that picture in my mind. It's not so easily done.

*Blocks to Forgiveness*

Forgiveness and acceptance are difficult for me. It helps for me to keep in mind a few strategies that *don't* work:

- Positive thinking
- Adherence to extreme belief systems
- Intellectual forgiveness vs. heartfelt forgiveness and acceptance

**Positive Thinking:** It doesn't work to suppress your feelings of anger and rage against a situation or person that has treated you poorly; first you have to experience the feelings. You must absorb the negative hit and then let it go. Creating positive thoughts about whoever has wronged you won't work. Only by forgiving them or the situation can you move forward.

Part of this aspect of dealing with anger is accepting at a deep emotional level that the pain you feel today is the pain you will have, in some form, for the rest of your life. Acceptance of this fact is the starting point in dealing with your pain-related stress reactions.

Letting go of positive thinking allows you to regain your life perspective. Many people in pain get caught up only in finding a solution. So when I ask my patients, "How are you going to live the next thirty or forty or fifty years with this pain?" they wake up. They've usually been bounced around the medical system without any coordinated plan, sense of control, or hope. They are so (legitimately) frustrated that they don't realize they need to look at their lives differently.

One patient, Alan, started undergoing various orthopedic procedures at age forty. His first spine operation was a laminectomy, removal of a bone called the lamina, which protects the back part of the spinal column; and then he had a fusion performed for back pain. Over a nine-year period, his spine broke down above and below the fusion. When he saw me, he was tilted forward about 30 degrees and tilted to his right side about 40 degrees. He had to use a walker. In the interim, he'd had both hips replaced, four knee arthroscopies, and both shoulders scoped. He felt pain throughout his whole body. Surprisingly, on his initial intake questionnaire, he rated himself as a zero on a scale of zero to ten regarding anxiety, depression, and irritability. He was clearly trying to use positive thinking.

I performed major spine surgery and corrected Alan's posture, for which he was extremely grateful. But he had a rough recovery in addition to his usual pain. He continued to deny any stress issues, though, and I could not crack his armor. It was clear to me how frustrated he was with all of his orthopedic limitations at so early an age, but I couldn't persuade him to do any writing or engage with the pain psychologist. About once every four visits he would get close to exploding, but then stuff it. He had an extraordinarily engaging personality and was seemingly happy. There was always a big smile on his face and I enjoyed his visits.

I never did get through to Alan. He continued to experience chronic pain and, shortly after I was through seeing him, underwent a total knee replacement. It is documented in the literature[5] that if you are not connected to your emotional pain it will be physically manifested in another part of your body.

If you are in chronic pain and haven't been given any answers or direction from the medical establishment, but really, truly, do not feel any anger, put on your gloves and start digging through your positive thinking veneer.

**Extreme Belief Systems:** Common mechanisms used to deal with anxiety are rigid thinking, control, and over-dependence on structure. These methods become apparent when anyone tries to control people and circumstances at home and work so they don't have to feel any anxiety about future outcomes. Anyone who does this is focused on their own opinions and probably not aware of the needs of those close to them.

For instance, a parent might criticize his son for being lazy for not doing his homework, when the real problem is that the son is upset about his relationship with his girlfriend.

Extreme belief systems fall into this category. They can be in almost any arena, including religion, politics, and nationalism. In this scenario, you become attached to being right. What you may not realize, though, is that this attachment is really thinly disguised anger, even if you don't consciously feel angry. Watch your reaction when someone disagrees with or questions your belief system; it will be an angry one. Someone merely disagreed with you; you weren't physically threatened or harmed. Why would you become so reactive?

I have deep respect for any person's religious or political beliefs—that's not the issue. It's the consequences of hiding behind them that concerns me.

Among the patients I've seen who cede the solution for their chronic pain to a rigid religious code, I've never witnessed one improve his or her life, function, or pain. I've tried everything from a full-on frontal assault to using logic, but I cannot get through.

A deep spiritual connection to yourself and a higher power can be conducive to healing. I fully support developing a deep, genuine faith, and many of my patients have had great success with the support of their religious leaders and fellow believers. However, any religious belief system that is critical of one's self or others is damaging. I cannot penetrate these patients' rigidity and have learned to let go, quickly.

**Intellectual Forgiveness vs. True Acceptance:** I was raised in a fundamentalist church that taught that forgiveness is the essence of life. Yet at the same time many religious cultures are intolerant of other belief systems. I still have many friends in the church community and I have a lot of respect for faith. But how can you be truly forgiving and judgmental at the same time? True forgiveness is a critical part of living a full, rich life connected to your family and friends. That said, I know that reaching that point at an emotional level is challenging.

Some consider certain acts unforgivable. (Imagine, for example, surgery that disables you for life.) I once would have agreed with that notion. In the past, I felt that forgiving certain deeds would be like denying they'd happened. And I still think that there's a fine line between forgiveness and acceptance, and denial. I now realize, however, that it's critical to forgive, regardless of the extent of the misdeed. The only one who will continue to suffer is you.

You can learn forgiveness from many sources. Commit to finding out which tools are the most useful for you and practice them. Repetition makes a difference. Learning to forgive may be the one step that most impacts your capacity to enjoy your life.

### *Reprogramming*
### Step 6: Play

A few years ago I was reflecting on my own journey out of NPD, thinking about what the next phase would look like. Recognizing that play pathways, like pain pathways, are permanent, I realized that the mental distinction between work and play was arbitrary. It was then that I decided to simply have a better time at work. I enjoyed my staff and patients more. I viewed the hassles and politics as just part of the job.

I think that play is the most powerful way out of the Abyss. It is a complex, creative pursuit that lights up an immense part of your brain. As your brain is engaged in this degree of widespread and stimulating activity, the pain pathways will quickly become uninteresting and eventually, dormant.

Playing with your family is an activity you may not have considered for a while. We get used to being in survival mode, and playfulness and creativity disappear. What can you do on a daily or weekly basis to create a household that everyone looks forward to hanging around in? Are you treating your friends better than you treat your family? Are you critical of your family? What gives you the right to be that way? If you met your spouse or partner today, would you act the same way you do right now? Is it important for you to be attractive to your spouse or partner? Are your children excited to see you or are they on edge because they don't know what to expect? Play will defuse the energy behind these questions.

Play is critical to pulling you out of the social isolation that so many of my patients experience. There are hundreds of research papers looking at the effects of social isolation. It is devastating. It's a catch-22 in that you don't feel like going out with your friends and you may not be the best company. That gives you even more time to think (obsess) about your pain, making it worse. Purposefully re-engaging with friends and getting out of the house is another effective way to leave your pain pathways.

## Stage 2: Forgiveness and Play—Final Thoughts

In Stage 1 of the DOC process, the basic tools of creating awareness, separation, and reprogramming are expressive writing combined with active meditation. Stage 2 is more complex, combining forgiveness and play. Both are involved processes that engage much of your brain. Humans evolved by interacting with other humans, and both forgiveness and play represent deep interactions with others. As powerful as they are in allowing you to enter a new life experience, unwillingness to engage with them will keep you pinned against the proverbial wall. I have long said that processing your anger is the continental divide of successfully solving your pain. Anger disconnects; play connects.

Stage 2 Suggested Reading
- *The Way to Love* by Anthony de Mello
- *Forgive for Good* by Fred Luskin, PhD

---

# CHAPTER 12

# Stage 3—Moving Forward

YOUR SUCCESS IN BECOMING AND STAYING PAIN-FREE depends on continuing to engage in the practices from Stages 1 and 2—the ones that helped you reprogram your brain and let go of anger. When you feel better, you may want to stop, but it's important to use the tools on a regular basis, indefinitely. Develop a doable set of actions in the early months, and then build on them.

A regular routine of action steps gets you ready to move on to Stage 3, where you consolidate your gains, develop organizational skills, and regain control of your day-to-day life.

## Five Steps

Step 1: Commit to a daily practice

Step 2: Create a safe haven—family

Step 3: Get organized

Step 4: Connect with the life you want

Step 5: Create your vision

### *Step 1: Commit to a Daily Practice*

Repetition is the key to reprogramming your nervous system. We all know how difficult it is to keep New Year's resolutions. Why? We are often quite serious about it at the time. But as the saying goes, "The road to hell is paved with good intentions." Researchers have long studied why it's so difficult to change behavior.

In one weight-loss study the participants who were successful in losing the desired amount of weight were the most likely to revert back to old patterns of behavior and regain the weight.[1] Even tasting success was not enough to sustain change. Behavioral patterns will win out unless you steadily chip away at them. So instead of having a broadly defined goal such as, "Get my life back," commit to specifics that are doable, and realize that you will frequently fail.

As you practice strategies that change the structure of your brain, you will notice your behavioral patterns evolving as well. Although you can't fix yourself, you can become an observer of your own healing.

I have learned to commit to small practices that eventually have made a significant difference. I am able to do my expressive writing at least one minute once or twice per day. I engage in active meditation as often as I can remember to do so, which is about five to ten times per day. There are several small inspirational books I look at for a couple of minutes, three or four times per week. I am committed to being aware of when I play the victim (often in creative ways), and this awareness allows me to re-direct my energies. I practice being grateful for what I have; just reading history or the newspaper helps remind me how lucky I am. I work out at the gym three or four times a week. Sleep is my greatest challenge.

By using these strategies, my behavioral patterns have changed. The small practices listed above allow me to engage in more complex strategies such as deeper acceptance, play, creativity, and giving back.

If I quit my expressive writing, I have recurrence of physical symptoms within a few weeks. My feet burn, my ears ring, I sleep poorly, I am more reactive, small skin rashes appear on both of my wrists, and I wake up with a headache. This is just the beginning, and other old symptoms emerge quickly. When I finally wake up and re-engage, I feel much better within a few days.

## The Power of Commitment

When I think of commitment, one event comes to mind. On Christmas Day, 2008, I was skiing with my son, Nick and his friend Holt. The three of us were standing on top of a cornice at Snowbird, Utah. For you non-skiers, a cornice is a steep drop-off of ten to twenty feet that forms from the snow being blown up the mountain. Most skiers make a diagonal trail down this drop-off, which is fairly safe. U.S. ski team-level skiers (like Nick and Holt) usually jump straight off them.

Below the cornice was a chute that was approximately twenty feet wide at the top but only about six feet wide two-thirds of the way down. About a hundred feet below us on the left there was an outcropping of rocks that stretched for two hundred feet. As Holt was figuring out his line I said, "Holt, I don't think your coaches would be thrilled with you skiing down this chute." He looked at me and immediately jumped into it. He skied about seventy-five feet straight down, made a gentle turn to the right, another gentle turn to the left, and ended up in a large bowl. Nick started off to the right and jumped in from a fifteen-foot cliff, making the same turns. They were each traveling over fifty miles an hour when they reached the open bowl. This was simply an undoable feat for most humans. If they'd hesitated midway—if they hadn't remained committed to their decisions—they would have run the risk of serious injury. Mind you, Nick's and Holt's certainty came from hours upon hours of practice over many years.

Commit to scheduling time daily for tasks you can accomplish; this will stimulate your brain to change. Eventually, functional behavioral patterns will emerge that will become your baseline. Don't hesitate in your pursuit of your new life—commit to yourself and your new reality. Life is short.

### Step 2: Create a Safe Haven—Family

Pain equals frustration. With chronic pain, frustration is intense and you will disconnect from your immediate surroundings. Your awareness goes to zero, which leads to abusive behavior. You may not consider your behavior abusive, but your family may see it differently.

When you're angry, your kids, spouse, or partner—who are dependent on you—have no control and become fearful. At a minimum, you cease to be a source of peace, joy, and happiness within your family or close support circle. It's likely you're not volunteering to be your kids' coach or taking an active role in their lives. Chronic pain takes a terrible toll on those close to you. Here are several suggestions for fostering healthy, loving interactions with family members and close friends:

- Read *Parent Effectiveness Training* by Thomas Gordon.[2] This classic has had a big impact on my life. Read it even if you don't have children. It will increase your awareness not only of your children's needs but also those you work and live with.
- *Never* engage with your family when you are angry. Wait until you are completely calm.
- Ask your family what it's like to be around you when you're upset.
  - Write their answers down and look at what you've written, or bring it to mind whenever you're tempted to interact with any of them while you're angry.
- Listen to your children without giving advice or an opinion unless you're asked. (This action step is courtesy of Hyde School.)[3]
  - I usually ask my patients to commit to doing this for a month

to begin the process. It should evolve into a lifetime habit.

- Work with all members of your family to create a vision of what they'd like their family life to look like.
- Institute a tradition of having a family meeting with an agenda once a week. (Hyde School again.)
  - You need your family or close circle of friends for your support. Don't become a living weapon with them as your target.

## *Step 3: Get Organized*

To stay on top of your goals and your treatment plan, it's important to be organized about it. This involves checking everything weekly and updating as needed. You may think that you're not an organized person and there's nothing that can be done to remedy it. That's not true: getting organized is a learned skill.

Organizational skills have never come easily to me, as I have a severe adult attention deficit disorder (ADD). I have been legendary since high school for losing things. I functioned well in medical school and residency because of the inherently tight structure, but when I entered private practice, organizing my time and efforts instantly became much more difficult. There were so many things coming at me from so many directions. Part of my identity had always been, "I am just not an organized person," but that needed to change, and fast.

I picked up a book, *The Organized Executive* by Stephanie Winston, and was quickly able to put the principles she presented into practice.[4] My first focus was and still is to make sure that I follow up on every test I order on my patients and answer their phone calls. Over time I was able to keep up on almost everything I needed to do to provide good follow-up care; very few things fell through the cracks. I would not have figured this out without help.

Later, my brother encouraged me to look at an organizational system created by David Allen, author of the book, *Getting Things Done*.[5] Because he was my little brother, I didn't jump at his suggestion initially. However, I noted that by using Allen's precepts, he'd gone from middle manager at his company to vice president within three years. He's now a senior vice president. I finally read the book and a month later, went to a seminar given by the author.

I was blown away—Allen's concepts are brilliant. His core strategy is to define any task that takes more than two minutes as a project. Everything in your life is filed away in a simple enough system that it is easily retrievable. The analogy he uses is putting all of our to-do lists on a "hard drive." Most of us keep our tasks in our RAM (random access memory), which means it keeps spinning around in our heads. This not only ineffective; it wears us out. (And it also reinforces obsessive patterns of thinking.)

If you outline and organize all your projects, however, it's possible to stop thinking sequentially. Instead of waiting to accomplish what you want, you just have to figure out "the one next step." That is a David Allen term, which in and of itself has changed my life. He describes a weekly mind sweep, when you review what's on your  hard drive  and add items to your  to-do list. Using Allen's book, I have been able to accomplish things I never would have thought possible. For example, this book would not have been written without my understanding of his organizational strategies.

Getting organized in the context of your chronic pain problem accomplishes several things, including: 1) Enabling you to decrease your stress by gaining better control of your environment; 2) Clearing creative space in your head so you can better solve problems; and 3) Helping you to move forward on as many fronts as necessary.

There are many organizational systems. Do a little research and find one that is right for you. Then, do the following:

- Decide whether you want to implement the system on paper, or use a computer or your phone.

- Use it! Don't let yourself off the hook. It'll be easier with practice.
- Don't put anything on your to-do list unless you intend to do it. Leaving items on your to-do list will destroy the process.

### *Step 4: Connect with the Life You Want*

One of the final steps in resolving your pain is to reconnect with your vision and the best part of who you are. These circuits are far removed from the Abyss and when you plug into them, they will build on themselves. It does require a deliberate effort, however.

During the early years of the DOC program, I came to realize the importance of establishing a vision. During this period, I used to work with patients intensively to help them heal and, in many cases, go back to work. Returning to a job can be complicated, so I would talk to attorneys and employers, helping pave a smooth re-entry.

One patient I helped with re-entry was Ralph, a fifty-five-year-old laborer who I'd been seeing every one to two weeks for about a year. He was progressing reasonably well, and I'd spent some time calling his employer and arranging a graduated return-to-work program. When I called to let Ralph know the program was in place, he told me that he was retiring and that he'd never intended to return to work. You can imagine my thoughts at that moment.

Turns out, while Ralph hadn't expected to retire so early, once he was in pain, he didn't feel good enough to go back to his job. So he figured retiring was his only option. He thought the DOC project was too much work and didn't think he could handle it on an ongoing basis.

That's when it hit me: when you are deeply sucked into mental and physical pain pathways, you rapidly lose your perspective. Your brain is stuck on thinking about your pain and how to solve it. It feels like the rest of your life will be taken up by these thoughts, and as a result, your outlook on life is decidedly negative.

My thinking in this area suddenly crystallized: I couldn't just work with patients on healing; I had to work with them on widening their perspective so that they could see the possibilities for their own lives. Even though Ralph had made progress in resolving his pain, he was still so focused on it that he didn't have the energy to return to work.

My experience with Ralph was in 2002. Afterward, I began to have early and clear conversations with patients about the goals of our working together so we could get on the same page. I would have my patients create a vision of where they wanted to go. This allowed us to work as partners; I feel that it's the only way treatment can work well. What began to emerge was a much bigger role for connecting with your life outlook. Do you see your life as filled with possibilities or as limited?

Regaining your sense of purpose and life vision is extraordinarily powerful in moving you off of your pain circuits. Once you are able to connect with your life vision, you may falter, but you'll never permanently return to your pain pathways.

Here is an exercise for cultivating excitement about the future—one that I have personally found helpful.

First, find a quiet time and place where you can just think and possibly go into a meditative state. Think back to the time in your life when you were the happiest. Next, visually take yourself back there, trying to remember every possible detail about that era of your life. Remember:

- Dreams and goals
- Attitudes
- Friends
- Activities
- Feelings and emotions around specific events

Spend some time with this exercise and repeat it a few times. As you visualize and feel this time period, you will wake up that part of your brain. Later, you can develop a plan for bringing this feeling of joy back into your life.

### *Step 5: Your Vision—Ask Three Questions*

To come up with a vision plan, start by considering this analogy: running your life is similar to running a business. While this may seem impossible in the context of chronic pain, there's no time when it's more vital. There are multiple components in your life that have to come together in order for it to be successful. You must assess where you are, envision where you want to go, and plan on how you are going to get there.

Where Am I?

Figuring out where you are is critical. To answer this question in terms of a business, you would start by assessing your current skills and assets. In the context of chronic pain, this step entails gaining an understanding of your problem and what you can do about it.

Start by outlining the important areas of your life (see below). For each of these areas, assess in writing 1) your current situation and 2) the tools and resources you have to overcome any obstacles. For example, tools you might consider using are expressive writing, an on-line course, or regular exercise. Resources could include access to counselors, physical therapists, or a good friend,

- Health
    - General health
    - Chronic pain
- Family

- Friends
- Work/career
- Hobbies/recreation

## Where Do I Want To Go?

Now that you've assessed where you are, it's time to figure out where you want go—this is your vision. The answer to Question #2 has to be specific. Responses such as, "I just want to get rid of my pain" or "I just want my life back" are not helpful because they're too broad. As you contemplate your answer, think about whether you want to regain your previous direction in life or establish a new one based on your current situation. If you continue without a compass, you are giving your life over to your pain.

You may feel you have a hundred excuses not to do this, but when will there be a better time? When is your life going to get easier if you don't take control of it? Find a quiet place and take a day to relax and consider your life. Take a mental tour of all of it. Then recall the exercise in Step 4 where you remembered the happiest time of your life.

Don't start developing your vision until you can regain the feeling of what life was like when you were actively pursuing your dreams. Be honest with yourself regarding all of this. Did you ever have dreams? Did you ever try to make them a reality?

- Once you've recalled a joyous period of your life, sit down again and compare it to the present.
- Visualize the contrast between your current life and that happiest period.
- Note the gap between the periods.
- Make a commitment to pursue your dreams or passions.

- Write your vision in as much detail as you can. Try to stay connected to the feelings you experienced in Step 4. This is not a writing exercise that you throw away.

After you've taken time for reflection, write down your vision without taking your pain into account. Think about how you'd like to live a fulfilling and enjoyable life in each of the areas from Question #1 (health, family, friends, work, and hobbies).

## How Do I Get There?

The next step is to develop a personal "business plan." Think about the short- and long-term goals you'd like to achieve. As with any business start-up, you're more likely to succeed if you have an actionable written plan, and the more specific, the better. See the self-inventory template in Appendix B for help with this task.

Create your plan, including actionable items in each category. Under "Health: chronic pain," create a detailed plan that addresses each area of the DOC program:

- Sleep
- Medication management
- Goal setting
- Education
- Stress
- Rehabilitation

You probably won't be able to create your detailed plan in one sitting—in fact, it might take a few months. But what else do you have to do that's more important than taking charge of your life, including treating your chronic pain? In the course of this process, you may discover that most of your energy has become consumed by pain instead of experiencing life.

## Get Happy Now

In answering the three questions above, keep in mind that it's common in our culture to feel that if you had more of "X," then you would be happier. "X" can include more money, better-behaved children, a nicer boss, etc. It can also include less pain. I don't disagree that good circumstances are better than bad circumstances. However, many circumstances are beyond our control. In Eastern cultures, it's often the other way around. If you can first attain peace of mind regardless of your circumstances, then you will have the energy to create the life that you want.

It borders on insanity to think enough variables could line up for you to be perfectly happy. Blame it on our culture, which drives us hard to achieve this utopia. But your peace of mind cannot be dependent on your external circumstances. Trying to control everything is a waste of the emotional energy you need to create the life you desire.

## Stage 3—Moving Forward—Final Thoughts

You cannot take control of your life without a plan and the skills to execute it. View this as a step-by-step process and proceed through each step. If you lack some of the skills, learn them. Getting back in control will decrease your anxiety and your pain.

Stage 3 Suggested Reading
- *Getting Things Done* by David Allen.
- *Parent Effectiveness Training* by Thomas Gordon, M.D.
- Goal-setting tools in *Back in Control,* Appendix B.

---

# CHAPTER 13

# Stage 4—Expanding Your Consciousness

LIVING IN THE ABYSS OF CHRONIC PAIN DESTROYS YOUR DREAMS and vision of what you feel might be possible in your life. The first part of your journey out of pain is to pull yourself out from the hole, but the real power lies within Stage 4, where you expand your consciousness and creativity. Your brain will respond with neuroplastic changes and create circuits that are incredibly enjoyable. Your pain pathways will weaken and be triggered less often. Your body will be bathed in reward chemicals such as dopamine and oxytocin and your nervous system will calm down. The more time you spend creating your big vision and regaining perspective, the better you will feel.

There are five steps in this final stage, Stage 4:

Step 1: Pass through the ring of fire
Step 2: Step into your new life
Step 3: Fail well
Step 4: Look up—your spiritual journey
Step 5: Give back

## Step 1: Pass Through the Ring of Fire

A few years ago I was introduced to the concept of compassion-fo-cused therapy (CFT), popularized by Paul Gilbert, at a conference on compassion. The speaker was a London psychologist, Dr. Chris Irons. He pointed out that there are three core categories that allow us to function as humans:

- Doing and achieving
- Threat and self-protection
- Contentment and feeling safe

He presented a slide that showed how people go back and forth between these three states. I was excited about the conceptual model and showed it to my daughter, who was in her early twenties at the time and wise beyond her years. She looked at it for a while and said, "These should be in circles." After some thought, I saw her point. Picture a circle with two progressively smaller ones inside of it. The outer ring represents our "doing and achieving." The middle one is "threat and self-protection" and the center circle is "contentment and feeling safe."

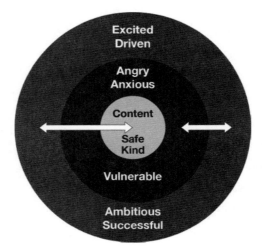

Many of us spend a lot of time trying to stay out of the middle ring of angry, anxious, and vulnerable by living in the outer ring of excited, driven, ambitious, and successful. It takes a tremendous amount of effort.

The outer level is a critical part of the human experience, and we go there when we engage in new activities, create new projects, meet new friends, etc. But living there exclusively is bad for our health—it involves a frenzy of activity and developing a façade to present to the world (and ourselves) that doesn't include having anxiety. Eventually, your activities, accomplishments, and possessions become your identity.

Many people can live their entire lives shifting between the outer and middle rings. It becomes more difficult over time, though. Most of this group eventually wears out, spending more and more time in the middle ring of fear and anxiety.

There are two ways to enter the center circle. The first is to expend your energy to the point of breakdown, descend through the "ring of fire" to your lowest point (the Abyss), and eventually end up in the center. You have heard the phrase that "people won't change until they hit bottom." When you have nowhere else to go and you are quiet enough to listen, deep change is possible. This is not the recommended way of finding your center, but it is the way I found mine.

I was raised in the middle zone. My family situation was difficult, filled with anger. As the oldest of four children, I spent an inordinate amount of my childhood trying to create calm, to no avail.

At age fifteen, I made a decision to live my life in the outer ring. I quietly shut the door on my past and moved on—except I didn't, really. I now know that my "moving on" was actually something called dissociation, where you disconnect from your true self. I suppressed the craziness of my childhood, created a life and persona that I wanted, and pursued my dreams. Sounds pretty reasonable, right? I was athletic, social, smart, and developed leadership skills. I took extra college credits in addition to working ten to twenty hours a week. I was having a great time experiencing this new life. I also developed an identity of being steady as a rock and cool. Nothing phased me or stopped me. I never got angry, and thought anger was a waste of time. I was somewhat legendary with regards to how much stress I could take for how long. Life in the outer ring was great.

When I entered medical school I developed another identity of "being compassionate, wise, and a good listener."

I became so enmeshed in the process of making over my life that my entire identity became the outer ring. For many years I was successful, or at least it felt like I was. The energy of my youth kept me hovering above the middle ring and I didn't even know what the word anxiety meant.

It worked great until I developed a severe neurophysiologic disorder that included relentless anxiety, progressing to a crippling case of obsessive compulsive disorder (OCD).

By 2002, I'd tried every possible means to pull myself out of my OCD, to no avail. I didn't realize that by spending so much time trying to both treat and avoid anxiety that I was actually fueling it. I was convinced I'd tried everything, and failed, so I had no idea what direction to go in. I was suicidal.

At that point I was completely stripped clean—every link to the identity that I'd created was broken. I had no choice but to question my entire belief system. That questioning resulted in me connecting to my anger. As I dealt with it, I inadvertently ended up in the center.

I now live much of my life in the center and am quickly aware of when I'm in the middle ring. I go to the outer ring fairly often, which requires passing through the "ring of fire" in the opposite direction. Any new endeavor, pleasant or not, creates anxiety. However, since I'm not unnecessarily burning my energy by avoiding anxiety, I can pass through the ring quickly. It was challenging at first, but got easier with practice.

I'm not happy about how I found my way to the center; I don't believe it's necessary to endure the extreme suffering I experienced to find it. My guess is that many of you are where I was—spending a lot of time trying to stay in the outer zone and spending too much time in the middle one.

You can start making your way to the center by developing your awareness. Once you become aware of which ring you're living in and have learned the tools to process stress, you have choices. You can choose to stay between the two outer zones, or pass through the "ring of fire" (middle zone) to the center. This means dealing with and facing your anxiety, which is a daunting prospect, I know. But if you use your tools to face your fears, it's possible, and not as difficult as you might think. It's infinitely easier than going down in flames.

The center is peaceful—I'm not constantly striving, nor in a constant mental frenzy. I am aware when I move out of it, and I use the tools that I learned to return to it. I have almost an endless amount of emotional energy and am limited just by the hours of the day and getting physically tired.

One insight that helped me understand the three zones was my tendency to procrastinate. I realized that it was associated with fear of failure or of rejection—the middle zone. The longer I put off a given project, the deeper the feelings. I tried to will myself to do better in this area—I made to-do lists and set deadlines for myself. But the fear was too strong and encompassing. I still got a lot accomplished, but continually charging through the middle ring by sheer force of energy wore me down. When I learned to become more comfortable with anxiety, I was able to start—and finish things—more readily. I still procrastinate sometimes, but when I do so, I use the DOC tools to work through it.

## Step 2: Step into Your New Life

Pursuing your real interests, based on your value system and sense of purpose, is what I call "living an engaged life." The intent is not to be perpetually happy—that's not realistic. Most significant pursuits involve challenges. But when you are connected to your real, authentic self, you feel greater satisfaction with success and possibly greater disappointment with failure. But you know that both are inevitable and you are OK with either.

Living an engaged life starts with gradually becoming more functional and shifting your focus from your pain to more interesting activities. It's much like what happens on your drive home at the end of the day. As you drive, you see many cars, houses, and trees, but your brain won't remember each one you pass; instead, you unconsciously screen most of it out because your nervous system is hierarchal. In other words, it remembers only what's most prominent. As you get further along in the healing process, your focus will be diverted from your pain onto your life—that is, the pain circuits will move down the chain in terms of your attention. The enjoyable activities you do will start to outrank your pain. This is why rehabilitation physicians emphasize function over pain relief in their treatment of chronic pain. If you assume that you have to get rid of your pain before you can live your life, forget it, you're done. Your pain will progressively occupy more and more of your conscious thoughts.

Along these same lines, if you're engaging in activities only to distract yourself from your pain, you'll have the same problem. Your pain will still be running the show. Do activities simply because you enjoy them and because they help you live a full and balanced life: don't hold on to any alternative agenda.

### Take Care of You

We can't change or fix other people—this idea has been around for a long time. It has been challenging for me in that from the time I decided to become a physician, my energy was focused on fixing people around me. In retrospect, I realize that I was focused on others, both to divert attention from myself and also in an attempt to save others to save myself. Of course, I didn't perceive that I, personally, needed any work at all. I was the healer. It was only under extreme stress that my façade finally crumbled.

The key to any success I've had helping others has stemmed from me being more connected to myself. I can talk to others on a human-to-human level instead of doctor-patient. I think that interaction may wake up the part of them that they have disconnected from in the midst of their suffering. It is also one of the reasons I initially ask my patients to use the simple tools presented in Stage 1; I want them to quiet everything down. At some point, my patients figure out how to heal themselves. Once they calm down and reconnect with themselves, there's no stopping them. It's like opening the door of a wild animal's cage. I've learned to just give direction when asked and stay out of the way. Every human, given a chance, wants to thrive.

There's a tendency among my patients, as they begin to experience success with the tools in this book, to try to engage their family members in the process. Although I do strongly encourage both halves of a couple to engage, they each have to do it separately and of their own free will. Any energy focused by one spouse on the other's progress is counter-productive.

Here are a few guidelines for staying focused on your own journey, and not on someone else's:

- Become aware of any energy you spend on trying to "fix" those around you. Instead, commit to your own growth.
- Develop an awareness of your own shortcomings and learn to accept them.
- Read an excerpt from *The Art of Living*, which is the teachings of Epictetus, a Greek Roman slave and philosopher, as translated by Sharon Lebell. His focus is almost completely on the journey inward.[1]

## Step 3: Fail Well

We are on hard on ourselves. We dislike failure and mentally beat ourselves up for it. But keep in mind that failure is a "story", just like success—it's subjective. What you may think is a terrible failure may seem like no big deal to someone else.

I deal with this issue with my patients. They come to my office enthusiastic about the early improvement in their pain and some even become pain-free within a few weeks. The positive energy emanating from them is palpable and inspiring. This is great news, right? Right. But there's one catch—often they're so excited to be doing well that they don't leave room for failure.

So around this time I tell them, "I am sorry to be the bearer of bad news but you are going to go back into the hole. These emotional and physical pathways are permanent." I tell them this not to discourage them, but to help them be ready, psychologically, for the days when the pain comes back. They, like many of us, believe they can create a world for ourselves that has minimal pain and suffering. So when they "fail" by having pain again, they become even more upset than they might've been, had they accepted that pain is just part of life.

It's not helpful to fight a sustained battle against pain, trying to pretend you can conquer it for good. You will consume your life energies. When you are down, you are down, and it's important to be able to be okay with that. One metaphor that comes to mind is a bamboo grove being buffeted by a storm with high winds. The grove can't stay standing in the wind; it essentially lays down under the pressure of the wind and rain. When the storm stops, though, it immediately stands back up. Part of the DOC process is learning how to fail, and then using your tools to get back up quickly—just like the bamboo.

## Step 4: Look Up—Your Spiritual Journey

I define the spiritual journey as experiencing life from outside yourself. Gaining (or regaining) a larger perspective will lead you to lose your sense of self-importance and increase your awareness of others' needs. It's a conscious effort. Here are a few things you can engage in that will help give you perspective:

- Quality time with family and friends
- Spiritual organizations
- Good food and wine
- Energizing experiences
- Creative hobbies
- The arts

Any experience that involves actively broadening your life view will work. This is particularly true when you can share it with others. Passive experiences such as watching TV are fine for relaxation, but they won't help you achieve spiritual growth.

Imagine what form your journey might take and write it down. Then revisit it regularly.

## Step 5: Give Back

The final step of healing is giving back. The urge to give back grows out of empathy, which is an inherent part of the human experience. Empathy is the ability to see a situation through another person's eyes with an understanding of what it might be like to be in a similar circumstance. It's often accompanied by a desire to help out.

Once you've implemented the tools that will reconnect you to your "authentic self" (Hoffman concept),[2] you'll have the desire, energy, and ability to reach out to others. I've observed this happening in my patients and it has been my personal experience as well. Patients free of pain want to give back—and in a big way.

I have a few suggestions to help you formulate your own ideas about how to give back:

- Stay committed to your own journey
- Remain aware of the fact that aside from yourself, your highest priority is your immediate family
- Make a random list of ideas about giving back that are interesting to you and then:
  - Pick the top five
  - Prioritize them
  - Develop a specific plan for how you are going to make them happen
  - Do it!

> *We are what we repeatedly do.*
> *Excellence, then, is not an act.*
> —Epictetus

## Stage 4—Expanding Your Consciousness—Final Thoughts

By this time in your journey you may have realized that, like the rest of us, you are not perfect. You will always have some level of anxiety and anger; but as you learn to accept these emotions as part of life, they will exert less of an influence on you. Instead of only intellectually accepting your imperfections, you will increasingly embrace the fact that they are part of the human experience, and stop trying to fix them. The ultimate solution is to direct your energy outward and create the life you desire.

Stage 4 Suggested Reading and Resources

- *The Art of Living* by Epictetus, translated by Sharon Lebell
- Healers, psychologists, psychiatrists, seminars, church, etc.
- A somatic workshop such as the Hoffman Process
- *The Way to Love* by Anthony de Mello

# SECTION 4:
# CONTINUING YOUR JOURNEY

# CHAPTER 14

# Sleep

ADDRESSING SLEEP WAS INADVERTENTLY THE BEGINNING of the DOC project. Years ago, I happened to read *The Promise of Sleep*, an autobiography by William Dement, who was a physician at Stanford.[1] Dement pioneered the science of sleep; his groundbreaking work included the development of the sleep lab. Because of this systematic study, we now know that there are over a hundred verified diagnoses of sleep disorders. He drew attention to the fact that sleep is an often overlooked variable in health care, pointing out that less than 5 percent of physicians routinely address sleep issues. Unfortunately, fifty years later, sleep is still undertreated.

I read Dement's book shortly after I moved to Sun Valley, Idaho, where I was caring for all aspects of my patients' spine problems. I noticed that most patients in chronic pain were not sleeping. I took an aggressive approach with medications and had them return for frequent follow-up appointments until they were sleeping reasonably well. This usually was accomplished within three to six weeks. Until I started doing this, I didn't have any idea how much sleep affected chronic pain. I was surprised to see how much patients' moods improved even before there was a decrease in pain. Sleep continues to be the one variable that must be addressed before there is any meaningful improvement in pain. Lack of sleep not only increases the perception of pain, it also decreases coping skills. Once pain begins to improve, patients can begin to reduce their sleep medication dosages pretty quickly, and then go off them completely.

A large population-sampling study from Turkey demonstrated that patients in chronic pain had almost double the problems with insomnia compared to those without pain.[2] Conversely, insomnia also seemed to be associated with a higher level of pain.

The Turkish study didn't look at whether lack of sleep caused the chronic pain or the pain interfered with sleep, but other research has shown that insomnia does in fact induce chronic pain. Another study followed more than 1,500 patients for almost four years. They discovered that there was almost a 50 percent higher chance of suffering from chronic pain with insomnia. The researchers looked carefully at the possibility of chronic pain being the cause of insomnia, but did not find any evidence.[3]

Many adults think they can get by on less than seven to eight hours of sleep, but that is simply not true. Consider seven to eight hours a minimum. An estimated 35 to 40 percent of adults don't get enough sleep, which translates into some type of sleep disturbance in over sixty million Americans.[4] You must be proactive in getting a full eight hours of sleep—allowing yourself to just lie in bed not sleeping night after night is unacceptable.

Addressing sleep is the first step—and an absolute necessity—in resolving anxiety created by chronic mental or physical pain. A recent study demonstrated that there is a higher correlation between disability and lack of sleep than there is between disability and pain.[5] The DOC program cannot be effective without adequate rest.

Here is a list of treatments for insomnia that should be implemented in a step-by-step manner:

- Sleep hygiene
- Bedtime stress management
- Exercise
- Over-the-counter medications
- Prescription medications
- Cognitive behavioral therapy
- Childhood trauma
- Sleep disorders

## Sleep Hygiene

Sleep hygiene is a term for a group of strategies used to improve the consistency of your sleep. Initially, in the context of chronic pain, these strategies often need to be supplemented with medications.

Some of the sleep hygiene[6] concepts are:

- Do not get into bed until you are ready to fall asleep.
- Watch TV, read, etc., in another room.
- Do not drink any caffeine after noon.
- Minimize alcohol intake in the evening—alcohol helps you to fall asleep but not stay asleep.
- Avoid heavy exercise in the evenings.
- Remove any clocks from the room. If you need an alarm clock, place it out of sight.
- Do something relaxing just before going to bed.
- Have a light snack if you're hungry.
- Concentrate on relaxing each muscle group in your body from head to toe. It is a form of mindfulness that switches your attention away from your swirling thoughts.

The older you are, the more important it may become to practice good sleep hygiene. The ability to get a good night's sleep takes a definite downturn around age twenty-five and a larger downturn at age forty-five.[7]

## Bedtime Stress Management

When you are under stress from either mental or physical pain, your brain is on a Formula One racetrack. It may feel hard to slow down your racing thoughts during the day, and next to impossible at night, in the quiet of your bedroom. A good part of this book is focused on stress management. As you more effectively process your stress, your sleep will definitely improve. As lack of sleep is, in and of itself, a major stress, this is a little tricky. Keep in mind that the combination of good sleep hygiene and medications can help you get better sleep, but understanding the role of stress in disrupting your sleep is important. Here are some suggestions:

- Don't read your emails within an hour of bedtime.
- Leave smartphones and laptop devices in another room and don't bring them to bed.
- Don't discuss controversial issues with your partner within a couple of hours of bedtime.
- Read a good book (in any room except the bedroom). A hard copy of a book is best, as the glow of an electronic device's screen keeps your nervous system stimulated. If you prefer e-books, there are devices and settings that can block the screen's blue light.

A 2003 research project assigned three different treatments to insomnia patients. One group was instructed to write how they felt in detail and to be really honest. The second group was told to write about activities that interested them or things they would like to do. The exercise was performed for a few minutes just before going to bed. The third group was just observed without any specific instructions. It turned out that both of the writing groups had similar outcomes, with a significant decrease in the time it took to fall asleep.[8]

Doing the writing exercises outlined in Chapter 10 is personally one of my most effective tools for falling asleep, whether at bedtime or if I wake up at 2:30 a.m. Keep a writing pad next to your bed so you can write if you wake up in the middle of the night; this will help you fall back asleep. It's remarkable how effective writing is in interrupting whirlpools of racing thoughts.

## Exercise

Regular exercise has been shown to have a modest effect on improving sleep. It can be aerobic, resistance training, or both. (Per the sleep hygiene principles, it should not be done in the evening.)

A systematic review paper from Taiwan demonstrated that exercise shortened the length of time needed to fall asleep, improved the quality of sleep, and decreased the use of sleep medications.[9] It is complementary to the other modalities for improving sleep.

## Over-the-Counter Sleep Medications

Medications are often needed for sleep when there's chronic pain. The first step is to try over-the-counter (OTC) sleep medications. These drugs are not primarily intended to induce sleep; instead, they usually have a side effect of drowsiness. For those with mild sleep issues, this can be enough to solve the problem with minimal risk. Here are some examples of OTC sleep medications:

- Melatonin: a chemical in your body that induces sleep. Rozeram is an example of melatonin in pill form that can gently induce sleep.

- Antihistamines: this category of meds has drowsiness as a side effect.
- Over-the-counter sleep aids: these are also mild with little downside risk.

With the exception of melatonin, the effect of these meds on the sleep cycle is unpredictable, but it usually takes about a week to find out if a given sleep aid is helpful. There may be side effects; for instance, some people who take them experience sleepiness the following day. If the drowsiness is problematic, it's best to switch to a different medication. A final note: OTC sleep aids can usually be safely combined with prescription sleeping meds. However, you must tell your doctor about of all the medications and dosages you are taking.

## Prescription Sleep Medications

If sleep hygiene, over-the-counter medications, and stress management have not been successful in helping you experience restful sleep, then it's time to work closely with your doctor to figure out which combination of prescription medications is best for you. Once you've started taking them, check with your doctor every five to seven days—either at follow-up appointments or via phone—to report how things are going. If the first treatment plan isn't working, your doctor should adjust it promptly, so that you're sleeping well within three to four weeks. This is the kind of aggressive, solution-oriented approach that I've found to be most effective.

If your doctor resists this kind of follow-up, don't back down. Calmly explain that getting sleep is a central part of your recovery program, one that you're taking seriously. Of course, if they still resist, don't be afraid to find another physician. (Note that some physicians, when dealing with sleep problems, opt for treating depression first, which does improve sleep. However, in my opinion, it takes far too long.)

There are several categories of prescription sleep medications, but they can classified into two basic groups, according to the way they work. One group directly induces sleep. The other group includes ingredients that are intended for other problems but have drowsiness as a side effect. Here they are:

- Sedative-hypnotics—intended to induce sleep
  - With anti-anxiety properties: Valium, Klonopin, Xanax, Halcion
  - Without anti-anxiety properties: Ambien, Lunesta, Sonata

The sedative hypnotic drugs with anti-anxiety properties shorten REM sleep, (rapid eye movement—the dream phase); whereas drugs such as Ambien and Lunesta preserve the normal sleep cycle. These drugs, with or without anti-anxiety properties, should be considered a short-term solution, as they can be habit-forming, and will eventually *increase* your perception of pain.

- Drowsiness as a side effect
  - Non-SSRI antidepressants: Remeron, Trazodone
  - Tricyclic antidepressants: Amitriptyline (Elavil), Nortriptyline (Pamelor)
  - Anti-psychotics: Seroquel, Risperdol

In addition to sleep medication, it can be helpful to take a slow-release narcotic, which will last for eight to twelve hours, to help with pain. I don't like using narcotics as a primary strategy for sleep, but they may lessen the pain enough to allow the sleep medications to work. (I will cover narcotics later.)

Another strategy for addressing sleep is to use anti-seizure drugs such as Neurontin and Lyrica, which stabilize the membranes of nerve cells. They seem to have a calming effect on the nervous system, and may improve burning nerve pain.

I won't go into the pros and cons of each medication—that is something to discuss with your doctor. Each physician will have a set of medications that they're comfortable with. Rest assured, you will able to find a combination that works. Pain is not a reason to lose a night's sleep.

It's not recommended to take prescription sleep medications without engaging in the rest of the DOC project. Long-term use of these drugs cause problems such as increased tolerance, dependency, more falls, injuries, traffic accidents, decreased cognition, and altered sleep physiology.[10] The intent is to provide you with some early relief so you can more fully engage in your healing and begin to break the insomnia/pain cycle.

## Cognitive Behavioral Therapy

Cognitive behavioral therapy (CBT) is a family of treatments that addresses maladaptive belief systems and helps shape your behavior to be more functional and appropriate in the situation. It may focus on some of the contributing factors to insomnia, such as anxiety and depression, or it can address maladaptive belief systems around sleep.[11]

CBT-Insomnia (CBT-I) is a problem-focused therapy intended specifically to improve sleep. You can learn more about it online, or a mental health professional can help you with this therapy individually or in a group setting.

*Bibliotherapy* is learning about a therapeutic approach from a book, and treating yourself. David Burns's book, *Feeling Good,* turned out to be the key to breaking me out of a fifteen-year tailspin of depression and chronic pain.[12] I happened to pick up his book in 2001 and ended up using it as a guide; his methods helped me to self-direct my CBT treatment.

CBT is effective through individual or group sessions. It can be taught by professionals other than psychologists, such as teachers, nurses, and physical therapists.[13, 14] It is important to realize that there is no standard CBT protocol, and indeed many different techniques are used to administer it. In other words, CBT is readily available to you without having to seek out a mental health professional.

## Childhood Trauma

While CBT addresses present-day beliefs that are disruptive to your basic well being, it doesn't dwell on past events. However, your past experiences also have an effect on your day-to-day reactions in a way that may increase your anxiety and disrupt your sleep. Therefore, it's important to become aware of these experiences. Looking at the past and CBT are complementary approaches to calming down your nervous system.

A landmark study performed on 17,337 members of the Kaiser Health Care System in 1998 divided childhood trauma into eight categories. They were termed "Adverse Childhood Experiences" or ACEs. The categories were:

- Emotional abuse
- Physical abuse
- Sexual abuse
- Household substance abuse
- Household mental illness
- Witnessed domestic violence
- Incarcerated family member
- Parental separation or divorce

Only 33 percent of respondents had an ACE score of zero, and 26 percent had an ACE score of three or more. People with elevated ACE scores, especially with three or more, had a higher incidence of depression, anxiety, severe obesity, suicide attempts, domestic violence, substance abuse, smoking, and increased risk of cardiac disease, among many other health problems.[15]

A difficult childhood has long-lasting mental and physical consequences that will affect a person's entire life, including sleep. It has been shown that insomnia correlates with an elevated ACE score: the higher the score, the more severe the sleep disturbance.[16]

Because these adverse experiences have an impact on brain development during critical formative years, addressing them is critical. This early programming is permanent, powerful, and solvable only by using strategies that stimulate neuroplasticity.

It is important to become aware of your ACEs because they determine your automatic reactions to stress. As you recall, the term for this phenomenon is "being triggered." When a current situation has a resemblance to a past trauma, your nervous system will react in the way it did when you were a child. You can't get rid of these triggers, but awareness will allow you to give yourself the space to substitute a more reasonable reaction. This process is best done with the help of a trained mental health professional, as you will need wisdom and support as you de-energize your triggers. One of the rewards will be a restful night's sleep.

Many people are afraid of addressing past traumas because they do not want to reactivate these feelings. But it takes far more energy to avoid them than to process them. I had an elevated ACE score of 5, and my experience was that dealing with my patterns was much easier than running from them. In retrospect, not knowing about triggers led to a pretty chaotic life, in that many of my reactions to adversity were out of proportion to the situation.

The penalty for avoiding these triggers is high; the resulting NPD symptoms can be disruptive and unpleasant (See Ch 4). And there are other difficulties; one study showed that suppressing thoughts or memories damages the hippocampus, the part of your brain that is responsible for sorting and retrieving memories.[17]

## Sleep Disorders

If the strategies in this chapter do not help your sleep within a reasonable period of time, you should get further testing by a sleep specialist to establish a firm diagnosis. There are over a hundred sleep disorders, restless leg syndrome and sleep apnea being among the most common.

Many of these disorders are treatable. For example, anti-Parkinson's drugs can be effective for restless leg syndrome. Sleep apnea, a life-threatening problem, is approached in a step-by-step manner, and often requires a continuous positive airway pressure (CPAP) machine. If left untreated, sleep apnea will adversely affect your cardiovascular system, since it robs your body of adequate oxygenation.

## Sleep—Final Thoughts

I am frequently asked to evaluate patients for surgery who have histories of chronic insomnia. They often tell me they've tried everything and still cannot sleep. Keep in mind that just as with solving chronic pain, there is rarely a single answer for inducing sleep. Every sleep problem is solvable with persistence and a combination of the methods presented in this chapter.

Restful sleep is the highest initial priority in your healing journey. The effectiveness of the DOC principles will be compromised if you are not getting seven or eight hours of restful sleep each night.

Pursue the above-mentioned steps until your sleep issues are resolved. Make it your responsibility to work with your primary care physician or rehabilitation physician to get a restful night's sleep regularly. Not one major decision regarding your spine care should be made until you feel rested during the day.

# CHAPTER 15

# Medication and Chronic Pain

MOST PATIENTS WHO ENGAGE IN THE DOC PRINCIPLES will experience a significant drop in pain, anxiety, and anger. Their lives re-expand, and they are able to decrease the amount of medications they are taking.

This chapter presents an overview of my approach to medication management. It's only my perspective and is not intended to be used as a standard of care. Each physician becomes familiar with his or her own repertoire based on experience. This holds true regarding not only the choice of medications but also the combinations and how they are dosed. My intent is to give you a feel for how you might view your own medication use and be able to have constructive conversations with your treating physician. Here are some of my observations:

- Medications are a significant aspect of resolving your pain. However, I never prescribe medications unless my patient is engaged in some version of a self-directed structured rehabilitation program. My litmus test is whether a patient is willing to do expressive writing. With few exceptions it is the foundation and starting point of the DOC program.

- The total number of medications should be minimized. Each one has multiple side effects, which are compounded by the other meds. I frequently see patients who are taking over ten medications. I am not their primary care physician and cannot make any specific recommendations to my patients, but that many different pills in one day cannot be helping you feel that great. If you are on multiple daily medications, commit to forming a partnership with your doctor to figure out which ones you can stop taking.
- The intention of the DOC project is to eventually have you come off *all* pain meds. However, this step is my last priority. As you feel better, you can take charge of weaning yourself off medications with the help of your prescribing doctor. Once you have established a partnership with your doctor, medication issues cease to be a major problem.
- The main goal of rehabilitation is to maximize your function with the limitations that you have. While short-term medications can improve a person's capacity to be more active, patients also need to put in a significant amount of effort. If they're not willing to increase their physical activity, then I can't be a prescribing physician. Medications are intended to assist you in increasing your function.

## Medication Overview

In my opinion, these are the categories of medications needed to adequately address the symptoms of chronic pain. In keeping with my belief that the number of medications should be kept to a minimum, I have limited myself to these groups:

- Narcotics (opioids)
- Anti-anxiety
- Sleep
- Anti-seizure/membrane stabilization

You might have noticed that I have not included a muscle relaxant category. Here's why: first of all, you cannot directly relax a muscle spasm with medications. Muscles can only be relaxed with modalities applied directly to the area, such as heat, ice, and massage. Muscle relaxants also have many side effects, although they do seem to provide some general relief. But since none of them were created for that purpose, I don't recommend taking them.

For the record, Flexeril (cyclobenzaprine) is a drug often prescribed as a muscle relaxant. Related to a family of antidepressants call tricyclics, one of its side-effects is drowsiness, so it is useful for sleep.

Soma, another muscle relaxant, metabolizes to a short-acting barbiturate, and is highly addictive. The benefit does not outweigh the risk.

## Narcotics (Opioids)

While I am not an advocate of long-term narcotics use, there is one situation where I think they may be useful within the DOC structure: when patients can't function at the most basic activity level. In this case, taking narcotics for pain can help significantly, although it does not solve the chronic pain problem. They may allow patients to move around more easily in the short term and start the recovery process.

Narcotics all have similar effects and side effects; they just vary in how they are administered, their potency, and their duration of action. In other words, codeine and oxycodone have the same effects and side effects, but oxycodone is much more concentrated.

Two basic categories of narcotics are: 1) either direct derivatives of opium or 2) artificially synthesized. Some direct opium derivatives include:

- Morphine
- Heroin
- Codeine

Examples of semi-synthetics are:

- Oxycodone (Percocet, Percodan, Tylox)
- Hydrocodone (Vicodin, Loracet, Norco)
- Hydromorphone (Dilaudid)
- Tramadol (Ultram)
- Methadone
- Fentanyl (Mylan)
- Meperidine (Demerol)

It's important to distinguish whether or not a narcotic is long-acting. Some are encased in a slow-release outer coating. OxyContin is short-acting oxycodone encased in a time-release capsule. It's critical not to chew a time-release narcotic or cut it in half—if you do so, the amount of drug ingested over a short time can be lethal.

Other narcotics are long-acting just by the nature of the drug's chemistry. The classic example is methadone, which has an extended duration. In fact, it lasts so long that if taken too often it can quickly build up and also become lethal.

### *The Downside of Narcotics*

I am careful about long-term narcotics, but not for moral reasons—I spent about five years prescribing them. Rather, I'm cautious because there's a significant downside. For one, there's the tolerance factor: the liver becomes more efficient in breaking down the drug and you subsequently need more of it to obtain the same effect. Secondly, many patients just don't feel that great on narcotics. They complain of fuzzy thinking, which they sometimes haven't even realized until they come off the drugs. Constipation is a problem that does not resolve with time and creates a lot of frustration. Thirdly, narcotics are addictive. If it's a true addiction, it's extremely difficult to break. Many times the line between tolerance and addiction is difficult—often impossible—to assess. Physical tolerance of narcotics is universal and not difficult to address. It's the psychological dependence and related behavioral patterns that are problematic.

The most disturbing aspect of narcotics is that they increase the sensitivity of the nervous system. The term for this process is "up-sensitization" or "opioid-induced hyperalgesia." In rat studies, it's been shown that repeated administration of narcotics causes the animals to be more sensitive to pain stimuli.[1] It's unclear exactly why this happens, but it may stem from the fact that narcotics cause changes in the glial cells in the brain and spinal cord, which insulate the nerve sheaths. I initially was skeptical of this problem but I've seen many patients feel better by lowering their narcotic dose.

Initially, I rarely stop or decrease a patient's current narcotic intake. Instead, we first deal with sleep and then stress—when you're in chronic pain, your life is difficult enough without the additional strain of coming off pain meds. Once you develop decent stress management skills, you can start a gradual tapering off of the meds. Any patient who has begun to taper his or her own meds will usually come off of them eventually. Having narcotics in your life is just not that great.

Dosage doesn't seem to factor in to patients' ability to wean themselves off narcotics. I have several patients who were on over 800 mg of Oxycodone discontinue their meds and go pain-free. They have also appreciated rediscovering the capacity to think clearly. Coming off of these medications when you're ready should be a goal of your healing process.

## Non-Narcotics
Anti-inflammatory medications such as ibuprofen decrease pain in two ways: by directly relieving pain and by decreasing inflammation.

Direct pain relief from anti-inflammatories works well and is predictable. Most of us have taken them for a headache, sore back, etc. Studies have consistently shown that they work as well as lower potency narcotics like Tylenol with codeine and Vicodin. What's more, a recent study of 336 children with arm fractures showed that the failure rate for pain control was 30 percent with codeine and only 20 percent with ibuprofen. In addition, the patients had fewer undesirable side effects with ibuprofen than with codeine. Both parents and their children were more satisfied with ibuprofen.[2]

Decreasing inflammation is a much different process than direct pain relief. An anti-inflammatory must be taken for at least two or three weeks for its full effect to kick in. Often patients find it difficult to sustain a pharmacological dose for the required period, and skip a day or two. But even missing a day will markedly diminish the drug's effectiveness. A few examples of anti-inflammatories include:

- Ibuprofen (Advil)
- Naprosyn (Aleve)
- Indomethacin (Indocin)
- Nabumetone (Relafen)

Tylenol, which is not an anti-inflammatory, is also an effective pain reliever. The drawback is that it has the predictable effect of causing kidney and/or liver failure if you take too much. It's recommended to take no more than four grams per day. And be careful—there are so many medications that have Tylenol as an ingredient that it's easy to inadvertently exceed this dose.

## Decreasing Anxiety

Anxiolytics (Valium-type medications) work very well for quick and significant relief of anxiety. That's the good and bad news. It's difficult to treat anxiety if you are consumed by it, so short-term relief from anxiolytics can be very helpful to get you started. The bad news is that they work so well that they are addicting. The addiction is not a true addiction; it's more of a dependency. In other words, you become dependent on the meds to allay your anxiety, which can flare up as you come off of them. So they are not the definitive answer and should only be used in conjunction with an aggressive program to treat anxiety.

## Sleep
Adequate sleep is necessary for you to solve chronic pain. Medications are often required, as was addressed in detail in Chapter 14.

## Drugs that Directly Affect the Nervous System
There are drugs that work directly on the nervous system by decreasing the excitability of the nerves. They were designed to treat seizures, but are also effective for nerve pain. Who responds is unpredictable but the relief can be dramatic. Since these drugs calm the nervous system they have some beneficial effects on sleep and anxiety.

Examples include:

- Gabapentin (Neurontin)
- Pregabalin (Lyrica)

## Depression
Antidepressant medications are effective in the short-term for treating chronic pain-associated depression. Many patients are so depressed and beaten up by their pain that they cannot move forward without meds. Antidepressants aren't a substitute for the work on stress management, however.

Some physicians address sleep by treating depression, which can cause sleep disorders. Others use the side effect of drowsiness in certain anti-depressants to directly induce sleep. Be clear of your doctor's intentions when he or she prescribes these drugs.

## Medication and Chronic Pain—Final Thoughts

With mental and physical pain impulses assaulting your nervous system, it's difficult to fully engage in the DOC program. Judicious use of medication for specific symptoms is an important and often necessary aspect of solving your chronic pain. The key to medication management is to never view the meds as the definitive solution to your pain, but as an adjunct to systematically addressing all variables that affect your pain. The ultimate goal of the DOC process is to become pain-free without medications and few physical limitations.

## CHAPTER 16

# Effective Rehabilitation

EFFECTIVE REHABILITATION IS A CRUCIAL PART of my patients' recovery, and it can't be effective without active, motivated participation. In this chapter, we will talk about the components of effective rehabilitation. I use the spine as the basis for discussion but these rehabilitation principles apply to any part of your body. Here is an overview of the principles:

## Begin With a Calm Nervous System

The first principle of effective rehab is that your nervous system must be calmed down before you start. If aggressive rehab is instituted before the nervous system begins to calm down, there is a significant chance that your will pain flare up. Pain is hyper-reactive to sensory input, especially in the affected area. Effective manual physical therapy usually requires vigorous soft tissue (muscles, tendons, and ligaments) and joint manipulation, and sometimes this modality causes more pain. This can be a problem for someone in chronic pain. Recall the experiment cited in Chapter 3, where a functional MRI scan revealed that the brain's response to a pain impulse increases 500 percent after being in pain for more than three months.[1]

If your nervous system is fired up, do whatever it requires to calm yourself down—including free writing and active meditation—before starting rehab.

## Choose Effective Physical Therapy (PT)

I have no personal expertise in physical therapy; I will only share what I've learned to expect from the practitioners I work with. I'm fortunate in that Seattle has a remarkable standard of physical therapy and most therapists have done advanced training.

I work with a few therapists regularly only because I like to communicate with them quickly about my patients' status and they know my expectations. They also tell me what is needed. I frequently quiz my patients about their experience. If a patient is from out of town, I'll often contact their local therapist to explain my patient's problem and share my thoughts. As a patient, one should expect a clear idea of what to expect and what is expected of you. One idea is to write down your PT-related questions and goals and make sure that these are addressed in your session.

Components of effective physical therapy:

- Careful assessment
- Patient education
- Advanced soft tissue and joint mobilization skills
- Specific and functional therapeutic exercise
- Long-term home-conditioning program

My goal in this section is to provide you with enough information in each of these areas for you to ascertain the quality of your care.

### *Assessment*

On your initial evaluation, your therapist should assess each of these factors:

- Posture
- Flexibility of your spine
- Tenderness of the soft tissues
- Flexibility of your hips, knees, and ankles
- Pain tolerance

If you are being treated for LBP, your therapist may treat only your lower back for a given acute episode, but this is an incomplete approach. Often there's a soft tissue and movement imbalance that needs to be addressed to solve the problem and prevent the symptoms from recurring. Following are some examples.

As your discs degenerate and collapse with age, you lose the reverse curvature of your lower back. This condition is called *lordosis*. Lumbar lordosis allows your head to stay centered over your pelvis, which minimizes the forces needed to stay balanced. As you lose this curvature, you may feel like you're tipping forward. The term we use for this problem is *flatback*. You can compensate for this imbalance in several ways. Walking with your knees slightly bent will allow you to be more upright. Your quads will quickly fatigue and the muscles in your lower back and buttock area will be forced to fire more than usual. The tissues in your groin will shorten and make it even more difficult to stand upright. A thorough assessment would include all of these factors.

The treatment would include stretching out the hips, mobilizing the spine segments to improve the lordosis, strengthening the buttock and trunk muscles, and calming down the inflamed tissues. If only the lower back was addressed, your symptoms would be recurrent and persistent. If your whole body's movement impairment is addressed, you have an opportunity to reprogram your brain to move without pain.

Another example is when the iliotibial (IT) band becomes inflamed. The IT band is a wide band of tissue that runs down the sides of both your upper legs. It connects the pelvis to the lower leg and is critical for balance and gait. Pain can be severe when it is inflamed. The pain path matches the one from the fifth lumbar nerve root, so it's possible to mistake tendonitis in the IT band for sciatica. Therapists with excellent soft tissue skills can usually tell the difference. Just pushing on this band and assessing the tightness and tenderness (instead of just assuming it's sciatica) will reveal tendonitis, which can be treated effectively in therapy. You may not need an MRI scan of your back.

I recall a situation early in my practice where I had evaluated a patient for low back pain; it was a soft tissue problem, and I prescribed physical therapy. On his return visit I noted that a lot of his pain was in his iliotibial band. I called up the therapist and asked why they hadn't treated the IT band tendonitis. The answer was, "You only wrote a prescription for us to treat the lower back." That was the last time I recommended that particular therapist.

Hip arthritis is commonly experienced as pain down the front of your thigh when walking. It's also the pain pathway for the fourth lumbar nerve root. Occasionally I discover that a patient sent to me for sciatica actually has hip arthritis. One patient I ran across many years ago had undergone four failed spine surgeries when the problem all along was hip arthritis. Putting the hips through a range of motion quickly reveals the correct diagnosis.

Hip arthritis also causes you to lean forward, and the patient may initially look as if they have a flatback of their lower spine. Again, treating the hip problem is the key to solving it.

A final example: I have seen several patients treated for a pulled hamstring when the problem was a ruptured L5-S1 disc. The misdiagnosis occurs because the first sacral nerve root (S1) travels down the area of the hamstrings. Palpating and stretching the hamstrings clarifies the diagnosis.

It's not your responsibility to figure out these diagnoses or pinpoint other factors that may affect your treatment and outcome; it's the job of your physician and therapist. I've included these examples to increase your awareness of what should be done to obtain an accurate diagnosis. If you feel you've only had minimal assessment from your health care providers, then talk to your physician or therapist.

### *Education*

For long-term success with your spine health, it's critical to become aware of all aspects of your care. A given round of physical therapy may solve a specific episode of back pain, but understanding the full extent of your problem will keep you from reinjuring the tissues.

Your education should include an overview of spinal anatomy provided by your therapist, a book, a website, or all three. The more visual the process, the better. By becoming comfortable with the basic language, you can communicate with your health care providers more clearly. Our hospital offers a "back school" regarding spine care, called "Back on Track." Groups of eight to twelve people meet with one of the physical therapists for two hours to discuss different strategies for safely performing daily activities. The goal is to learn by listening, doing, and asking questions. There's also a lot of sharing. Regardless of where my patients are receiving their physical therapy, I ask them to attend this class.

Feedback on the class has been uniformly positive. One long-term back pain patient markedly decreased her pain by changing just one activity that she'd been doing improperly.

Remember, discs normally degenerate with age. It's not a disease and has not been shown to be a source of neck, thoracic, or low back pain. A better term would be "normally aging discs."

I recall a sixty-year-old man who'd been experiencing back pain for about eight weeks. He was terrified because he'd been told he had degenerated discs. He feared paralysis and loss of function. I explained to him in detail that his spine was completely normal for his age. All of his discs had degenerated, but discs normally degenerate with age. Armed with that information, the man's anxiety lessened and his pain immediately diminished. It's common that just knowing the problem isn't serious will decrease your perception of pain.

The second educational step is to understand how these principles apply to you. Be specific with your therapist about what aspects of your lifestyle are potentially irritating to your spine, so that you can develop new behavioral patterns to avoid injury.

### *Advanced Soft Tissue and Joint Mobilization Work*

Manual therapists are physical therapists with advanced soft tissue training, often through a certification course or a residency program. You can ask what kind of training they've had—it should be extensive. More importantly, you can assess their skills by how aggressively and effectively you are physically being treated. If the treatment is passive, such as the application of heat, ice, or ultrasound, chances are they don't have advanced skills. The idea is to progressively stretch the tissues until they are back to full range, have normal tone, and range of motion. I routinely ask my patients what types of treatment their physical therapists are using.

When I first began my practice I spent some time with a couple of advanced manual therapists to see if I could improve my physical examination skills. I quickly learned that it was impossible for me to duplicate the sensitivity they'd developed in their hands after examining thousands of patients. It's an important skill, one that requires both training and experience to develop. I felt that manual therapy had some similarities to surgery in that regard.

With deference to the manual therapy experts, I have a basic concept of what they do, divided into two categories:

- Segmental mobilization
- Myofascial work
  - Directly around the spine
  - Surrounding soft tissues and joints

One vertebral segment is defined as two vertebrae and the disc in between. Most patients have five motion segments—that is, segments that move—in their lower back. A few people have four or six. A good manual therapist can feel how much a segment moves compared to the next one. The goal is to have all the segments move about the same amount. Therapists can also determine which segment is painful through palpation and symptom analysis.

In examining segmental movement, there are many possible combinations to be discovered. For example, four of the five segments might be stiff while the fifth moves too much, which implies that the more mobile segment is absorbing too much force. With repetition throughout the day, this hypermobile segment could become irritated, and so the idea would be to increase the motion of the other segments by manually manipulating them. You would then have a more even distribution of forces throughout all of the lumbar motion segments. (Also note that mobilizing all of the spinal motion segments requires a significant commitment of time and can be very painful.)

Another common situation is that all of the segments in the lower back are stiff. To my mind the solution to this issue is a little more debatable. If the whole spine is stiff and the actual segments aren't moving much, then the spine is less likely to be the source of pain. It's more likely that the pain comes from the supporting soft tissues around the spine. In this case, it's my feeling that you should try to increase the mobility of the soft tissues around the hips to allow more motion there, causing less motion and stress across the back. I realize this is my own view—and arguable—but I have seen improved hip mobility decrease back pain many times. Even when I perform a fusion of the entire spine from the neck to the pelvis, there's still some flexibility left; patients can still bend forward at the hips.

Next comes myofascial work. Myofascial is the combination of a muscle and the thin, tough layer of tissue that envelopes it, called "fascia." Muscles themselves do not contain pain fibers; it's the fasciae—or connective tissues—that contain an abundant number of them. The fascia is the layer that may become inflamed and painful.

With pain, there's an instinctive tendency to guard the injured area. As a result of chronic limitation of motion, the tissues will shorten. When you then try to put them through a normal range of motion, they will be painful, and remain irritated.

Myofascial work is focused on specific massage techniques to identify which structures are inflamed and shortened, and then stretch them out. As you might imagine, if you take an inflamed, shortened muscle and perform a directed deep massage, it can be a painful process. The pain can be decreased somewhat with ice, ultrasound, and some other modalities of physical therapy. Good myofascial work is going to be somewhat painful, however; there's no way around it.

In an example above I mentioned the idea of improving hip movement, which is necessary for any thorough back treatment. Manual therapy includes stretching and exercise of the hip capsule with large motions, and also working on specific tight myofascial structures around the hip. It also will include joint mobilization of the hip itself.

Practitioners spend years learning and perfecting these soft tissue techniques. I've provided just a few simple examples to give you a feel for the concept. It's remarkable to me how an excellent manual therapist can improve flexibility and decrease soft tissue pain.

Most chiropractors have expertise in mobilization and soft tissue techniques. They are also allowed to perform "manipulations," where a stronger force is used to put a given joint through a wider range of motion. They offer a variety of methods. I have worked with many chiropractors who have greatly helped my patients deal with non-specific low back pain.

Whether a therapist or a chiropractor performs the soft tissue and joint work, it's critical to combine it with the key components of education, assessment, specific exercise, and a long-term plan.

### Specific and Functional Therapeutic Exercise

Your physical therapy experience should include a specific exercise program to address the condition and length of your muscles, your mobility and strength, and your functional ability. A physical therapist is the best qualified medical practitioner to apply one of the most effective modalities for low back pain—exercise!

I have seen several patients who are significantly deconditioned after years of chronic pain become transformed through movement and exercise. Many times they are completely surprised at their body's exercise ability. Once these patients recognize their ability to move in a less painful manner and identify, along with the therapist, activities that will improve their conditioning and strength, I have seen terrific results. These are usually my most enthusiastic converts to a lifetime of exercise and activity despite their condition.

Many patients are understandably fearful of movement and exercise of the painful area because they are worried about causing further injury. Occasionally, cognitive behavioral therapy is needed to address the maladaptive thought patterns that arise out of the chronic pain experience. CBT also has been shown to improve engagement in a long-term conditioning program.[2]

With a chronic painful condition of any part of the body, deconditioning of the muscles will occur. It is up to your physical therapist to prescribe a progressive and appropriate exercise program to recondition your muscles, strengthen your limbs, and allow you to move in a pain-free manner. An effective program will include aerobic activity, stretching, strengthening, and coordinative exercise. It will be challenging and difficult to perform at times. Although it may be painful, it will not hurt you. You should be able to recover from the effects of any activity within twenty-four to forty-eight hours and not be in a worse state afterwards. If any activity increases your pain and dysfunction longer than that, you should tell your practitioner.

Early in my practice I saw many patients with pain in the middle of their thoracic spines. I ordered many tests and injections in my attempts to identify their source of pain. I do not think I ever found one. I did have access to a great PT, so I also had patients begin a workout program. I encouraged them to start with light weights and high repetitions and gradually increase the weights. They focused on moving the area that was painful. Essentially everyone who stuck with a program had the pain resolve over three to six months. There was also the added benefit of feeling better and energized by the exercise regimen.

### Long-Term Conditioning

Your physical condition impacts the quality of your life, regardless of whether you are suffering from mental or physical pain.[3] Exercise has innumerable benefits—it's invigorating, it improves your mood, it burns off stress. Not exercising means you miss out on all of this. If you're in chronic pain, why would you even consider expensive and risky treatments with known poor outcomes without covering this base?

You won't be able to sustain a long-term conditioning program without first looking closely at your own behavioral patterns. Your conscious brain will not be able to overcome them with willpower. Everyone knows it's important to get into shape. Why don't we do it?

I have a college classmate who is a nurse on a pediatric kidney transplant unit. She was talking about her experience regarding why these transplants fail. It's not from a mismatch of donor versus recipient; it's because patients don't take their medications. They are unhappy that they've been robbed of a normal childhood and just don't care enough to comply.

One study looked at a rigorous weight-loss program for adolescents. Many of them successfully lost weight, exercised, and felt much better both mentally and physically. Yet most of them stopped the program and regained the weight; even the ones who'd been most successful initially. The factor that correlated with the lack of ongoing effort was the ACE score. ACE stands for "Adverse Childhood Experiences," as discussed in Chapter 14. It was this observation that was the impetus for the ACE study.[4]

## Daily Care

The first part of any conditioning plan is to incorporate what you've learned from your physical therapist about posture and body mechanics into your daily activities. It's the most important step, taken to avoid reirritating tissues that you've finally persuaded to calm down. No amount of fitness will override continuing to place abnormal stresses across the painful area.

## Weight Loss

The spinal column is not well-designed for upright posture. Your upper and lower body are connected by one structure, your spine, that is inherently unstable. Without the support of your trunk muscles and the small muscles directly connected to the spinal column, the spine would buckle and collapse with only four pounds of force applied to it.[5] Trunk support consists of: 1) the abdominal muscles, 2) the abdominal contents, which are liquid and provide support (similar to the bladder inside of a basketball), and 3) the surrounding muscle groups.

Patients often tell me that if they could lose some weight that their back pain would improve. More often I have observed the opposite phenomenon. As my patients have lost weight, their back pain increases. This is likely because there's less tissue within the abdominal cavity for the muscles to compress against, and therefore less support. Don't get me wrong—I strongly favor losing weight. However, your priority should first be general conditioning and developing muscle tone. The weight will gradually come off without increasing your pain.

## Strength Training

Strength training is a major factor in reducing pain. I think there are several reasons. First, there is the obvious benefit of having more strength, so a smaller percentage of your energy is spent on daily activities. You are able to stay well away from the pain threshold.

Second, you also have the capacity to engage in more vigorous physical activities that are enjoyable, taking your attention off your pain pathways. Many of these activities can be with other people.

Finally, although it's not going to be at the level of a long-distance runner, there is some degree of endorphin response with strength training. (Endorphins and enkephalins are the body's natural pain killers.)

Overall, I think the most important contribution that strength training adds is the reprogramming function. You are now sending a different set of signals from the body parts that are normally firing pain impulses to the brain. As you are voluntarily stressing a given muscle group, you have control as to the intensity of the signals. Somehow the combination of control and different inputs has a significant impact on pain.

I recommend that all my patients (and their spouses) work out with weights in the gym three to five hours per week, indefinitely. Many people roll their eyes. You can choose not to work out, but know that it will be difficult to recover from your pain if you're out of shape.

It's been shown that people over forty-five receive a tremendous benefit from weight training. We all lose a certain percentage of muscle mass every year (estimated to be about 1 percent), so resistance training becomes more important as we age. With weight training, you not only prevent the loss, you can also significantly improve your strength. This is the reason I ask the whole family to participate in resistance training. Since life spans are more than thirty years longer in the twentieth century than in earlier eras, it means each of us will lose 30 to 50 percent more of our strength.[6] This is preventable with consistent training.

Regarding the workout program, essentially all of the machines are safe. Avoid free weights, as there is more risk. You should begin with using light weights and high repetitions of fifteen to twenty per muscle group. Avoid unsupported bending at your waist no matter what the situation. Supported bending is fine, and so is twisting.

Most health clubs offer at least one free personal training session to get you set up and to make sure you are safe. Many physical therapists will help transition their patients from the specific/functional exercise phase into a long-term conditioning program.

I prefer weight training to be done outside of the patient's home. Very few people will consistently work out at home. It's helpful to be in an environment where others are working out hard; also, the equipment is better. Pilates is also excellent in that it emphasizes core strength, and I think yoga can be helpful if the extreme postures across the lower back are avoided.

## Core Exercises

Core exercises emphasize posture and focus on the small muscles next to the spine. Training the smaller muscles helps coordinate the movement between the vertebral segments, making it less likely that one segment will become overstressed and painful. Physical therapists will train you to engage these muscles in combination with weight training and establish a pain-free movement pattern.

Good general core awareness, adherence to proper body mechanics, and conditioning with weights in the gym will maintain your spine health for a long time.

## Depression and Exercise

Research has shown that those who are depressed and catastrophizing are less likely to exercise and comply with care. In their frustration, patients understandably don't want to commit to working out; they want the easy way out, looking to outside sources to cure them. Thinking like this, however, is a passive way of caring for your health. It's not dissimilar to being markedly overweight and bemoaning your knee arthritis, hypertension, and diabetes. If you choose to remain passive about your health, that's fine, but you lose your right to complain about it. You also cannot expect the medical profession to make up for self-inflicted disease. Cognitive behavioral therapy, which is part of the DOC program, has shown to help improve compliance with care.[7]

## Physical Therapy—General Concepts
### *Demand the Best*

As you read this chapter, you might be thinking, "I didn't go through all that when I went through physical therapy." And most likely you also didn't get better. Although a lot of therapists in my area do cover all of these bases, there are also many that don't. When I have a patient with ongoing low back pain, I always ask what kind of therapy they've already had. Frequently I discover that it's been limited to some ultrasound, heat, ice, and/or light massage. Vital aspects of the process have been overlooked, such as an evaluation of pelvic girdle muscle balance or a discussion of any workplace or lifestyle demands on the back. I'll find out that there's no long-term plan in place.

If a patient in my care has had unsatisfactory therapy, the first step is to send them to a therapy group that *does* cover all the bases. That frequently solves the problem.

Why am I so demanding about asking for a high level of expertise from physical therapy? It plays a major role in your recovery from chronic back pain. Many patients who've had inadequate physical therapy services conclude that therapy has failed when, in fact, they haven't really given it a fair chance. They become frustrated at the lack of improvement and opt for surgery, when it may be unnecessary. The most common reason given for performing a spine fusion or inserting an artificial disc to relieve low back pain is failure of non-operative care. Considering the risks of surgery and unpredictable outcomes, this is a high-stakes game. At a minimum, you should have worked hard with a structured rehabilitation program, such as the DOC program, for at least 6 months.

### Desensitizing the Soft Tissues

There is one final goal of physical therapy that we will discuss here: desensitizing the soft tissues.

Soft tissues become sensitized—or overly responsive—when the nervous system is subjected to a chronic, repetitive stimulus. All the healing elements we've covered so far—improving sleep, dealing with anxiety and anger in a proactive way, cognitive behavioral theory, improving function, and substituting new circuit patterns for old— contribute to the desensitization process. The other crucial piece of this process is for your physical therapist to work directly on the soft tissues.

First let's look at how sensitization develops. Consider the cycle of pain that occurs when soft tissues are injured. First, there's the injury, which, when it occurs in the low back, is often dramatic and severe. The initial pain causes anxiety. Then the anxiety causes you to guard the painful area (that is, not use it), thereby making the tissues stiff. Movement exacerbates the pain and leads to more guarding, especially if the tissue is moved too quickly or with too much force. As the brain starts to focus on the pain, the pain circuits intensify, which again leads to more guarding and stiffness. Guarding typically lasts a few weeks and then resolves. If it continues for several months, however, the soft tissues won't move as easily or as well.

My patients find it difficult to understand that the pain can get worse without additional injury; guarding—an act people think protects their back—is actually one of the contributing factors. All soft tissue is protected by pain-inducing fibers that are stimulated when the physical limit of that tissue is reached. For example, take your wrist and bend it forward with your other hand as far as you can. What happens when you reach the limit of your flexion? It hurts. If you then try to push it further, it hurts a lot. Now imagine your wrist being in a cast for six weeks. Anyone who's lived with a cast knows that the worst part is taking it off because the joint is stiff and sore. If you were to repeat the wrist-bending experiment at this point, you'd only have to move it a third to half as much to produce the same pain response.

Physical therapists work to resolve pain by pushing the limits of the contracted soft tissues to allow a full range of motion before the patient feels pain. Stretching increases the tissue's flexibility, which then allows for more motion. Therapists take into account that the nervous system is overly sensitive, and so try to keep the pain caused by therapy at a tolerable level. They will do this with soft tissue and joint mobilization techniques and/or exercise. Gradually, with repetitive stretching and controlled stimulation of the nervous system, the pain will diminish.

## Excellent Rehabilitation—Final Thoughts

During the first few months of your healing, it's important not to get distracted by chasing every possible solution. Once you begin to feel better, you should gradually look at and address the following variables:

- Smoking
- Diet
- Weight
- Alcohol intake

When I was in the depths of my pain, I didn't have the energy to look at any of these variables. I just wasn't interested. Until you feel better, I think initially it's helpful to let these variables go, as you will burn up a lot of mental energy feeling you should be doing something you cannot accomplish.

As for exercise, one incident reminds me of its power. My father-in-law, who passed away at age ninety, started a vigorous twice-a-week gym program at around age seventy-five. When I asked him why he started his new regimen, he said that he simply wanted to add fifteen yards to his drive on the golf course. He also wanted to be able to play golf with his son. As a result of this commitment, he lived a normal physical life with few limitations. He played tennis twice a week and could hit a golf ball about 175 yards up to six months before he became ill. Why wouldn't you want to remain fully physically functional for as long as possible?

Aside from remaining physically fit for its own sake, think about how it will enhance your quality of life. If you're in chronic pain, chances are your quality of life is dismal. Exercise will improve not only your function, but also your outlook.

If you're contemplating surgery, think about the fact that spine surgery is unpredictable in resolving low back pain. Exercise is a much more reliable solution. You may be avoiding exercising because of your chronic pain, therefore becoming less physically fit. Being in bad physical shape leads to even more pain. That cycle is deadly.

I've spent a large portion of this book discussing how to calm down your nervous system. One benefit is that you have more mental energy to commit to exercising. Actively engaging in a conditioning program takes time, but also strength of mind. With a calmer nervous system, you will feel less pain and cope better with the challenges that do occur with physical therapy.

# CHAPTER 17

## Expanding Your Horizon

A MAJOR PART OF MY JOURNEY OUT OF CHRONIC PAIN was broadening my perspective so that I could envision the possibilities for my life. Once I had perspective, I was able to embrace my future. Keep in mind, perspective isn't something you gain and then never lose. I have to consciously work on keeping mine so that I don't fall back into the depths of the Abyss.

Here are some ways that I retain my broad perspective. This aspect of the journey is an individual endeavor, so you can experiment with these and see which one works best for you:

- Nurturing gratitude
- Reading history
- Exploring a spiritual path
- Active self-discovery
- Connecting with others

### Nurturing Gratitude

The book *The Art of Happiness,*[1] based on extensive interviews with the Dalai Lama, explores the concept that we compare ourselves to others whom we perceive as having more than we do and, as a result, feel frustrated and unhappy. "Why not compare yourself to those who have less than you and be grateful?" he asks. It may be because in our brain's default survival mode, we are always looking for danger. To be grateful requires a conscious effort.

Several of my life experiences have strengthened my level of gratitude. They were all close calls with death:

- A head-on 100 mph impact car accident on black ice
- Having my head brushed by a passing bus mirror in Florence, Italy
- An early diagnosis of esophageal cancer on a random biopsy
- My almost-completed suicide attempt
- Missing a telephone pole by five feet at 60 mph when my friend's car spun out of control on wet pavement

I don't think you have to have brushes with death to be grateful to be alive, but I suspect that if you think about it for a bit, you would come up with a number of close calls from your own life. I view every second of my life as bonus time and feel privileged that I'm able to give back to others suffering in pain. I still think it's the worst experience of the human existence.

## Reading History

Read any history of almost anything and it will—or should—wake you right up. There is nothing in our modern era to complain about, compared to the ordeals of the past. When my patients become stuck, I frequently recommend that they read about a major world event or watch a movie about it. One example is *Man's Search for Meaning*,[2]

Viktor Frankl's first-hand account of living in a concentration camp. Frankl was a Jewish Austrian psychiatrist who survived the horrors of Auschwitz, including losing his family. Astoundingly, he was able to find meaning in the midst of his extreme suffering. He kept asking the question, "What is life asking of me now?" It was eye-opening to me to realize that a human could think and feel at this level in this kind of environment.

Another book that made a big impression on me was *The Swerve* by Steven Greenblatt.[3] Greenblatt researched the discovery of an ancient Greek poem, *The Nature of Things*, written by Lucretius, and pulled the reader into the lives of people who lived in the Dark Ages. Our worst day ever is infinitely better than anything they could have imagined; in addition to random executions and torture, there was no medical care and the average life span was only about thirty years. When things get bad, I remind myself that I'm happy to be living in this era.

Somehow in the midst of our busyness we forget how most of the human race has lived and is still living in much of the world. There are an endless number of books that have had the same effect on me. Wake up! We are living in the most advanced civilization in history.

## Exploring a Spiritual Path
### *The Journey of 1,000 Moons*

One concept that I've found helpful to gaining perspective is a project called "The Journey of the 1,000 Moons," created by my friend, the artist Ernesto Sanchez. Here is Ernesto's description of it:

> *If you count the moon cycles you will experience in your lifetime, by the time you reach 77 years of age you will have experienced one thousand of them. As we live these years, how often do we stop and think about the role of the moon in our lives and on the earth?*

*To honor the inspirational force that the moon has on my life, I began an art project called "The Journey of 1,000 Moons." The goal is simple: to make 1,000 moons. The moons are cast in gypsum and hand-painted. Like our lives, each moon is unique. For every journey, there is a path, and on the path are points of inspiration, illumination, and revelation. But you cannot experience these unless you take the journey.*

*"The Journey of 1,000 Moons" reminds us that while the energetic dance between the moon and the earth has endured for billions of years, each of our individual lives is but a brief flash of illumination—only 1,000 moons.*

Ernesto's ritual "moon burning" ceremony—in which he burns one of his moon sculptures—can represent many things to the participant. For my patients there's the obvious metaphor of watching your life go up in flames living in chronic pain, or it can also symbolize letting go of your past and moving forward.

Ernesto has been an inspiration to me with his commitment to the arts as a way of elevating the spirit. This concept is helpful for me in the midst of the chaos inherent in being a complex spinal deformity surgeon. It can be used to bring balance to any chaotic life, including one that's touched by chronic pain. I have two of his moon sculptures hanging in my office.

How many more moons do you have left to see before you are seventy-seven? How much more of your life do you want to spend living the way you are right now?

## Active Self-Discovery

Use active self-discovery tools as an adjunct to the basic skills for addressing anxiety and anger. There are thousands of resources that provide tools to help you live a more satisfying life; this chapter touches upon a few of them.

While I do think that every resource I used in the past—books, practices, etc.—helped me in my own journey, one problem was that I was on an endless journey to fix myself. Whenever I found a new tool, I'd feel that it was the complete solution to all my problems and the key to transforming my life.

My belief that I could fix myself was derived in part by my poor stress management skills. I feel strongly that if I'd been taught stress management skills early on—in middle or high school—I would not have been on this quest. If I'd had the skills, I could have processed stress in a more constructive way. But instead of having the knowledge I needed to live a full, interactive life, I was always in survival mode.

### *The Hoffman Process*

The Hoffman Process is one example of a personal growth program that allows you to powerfully expand your consciousness in a short time. Hoffman-trained teachers explain how to break up entrenched neurological pathways and reprogram your responses to the events that trigger them. In other words, instead of experiencing stimulus, then response; the pattern becomes stimulus, then choice of response.[4] The tools this program offers help you learn how to break the compulsive link between any given situation and your automatic response. In my experience, reprogramming work which would take years on your own can be accomplished in seven days.

There's a strong connection between the Hoffman techniques and neurophysiologic disorder. The essence of NPD is that you have neurological pathways that will predictably become activated by a specific circumstance or level of stress. All of our responses to stress are essentially pre-programmed so that a specific stimulus will elicit a fairly predictable reaction. Any time you're anxious, you're probably in a "pattern." Hoffman helps you to break out of the pattern.

Hoffman is not for everyone, and it's also not within the budget of many people; but there are other programs and resources available that emphasize connecting thoughts with physical sensations. The term used to describe this type of process is "somatic work."

I would encourage you to actively pursue every avenue available to improve your ability to process stress. You'll connect with some and not others. All of it will be uncomfortable and some of it painful, but it will enable you to live a better, more satisfying life.

### Psychotherapy/Counseling

At one point in my life I thought that traditional psychological counseling was the only way to deal with stress. Then I became focused on cognitive behavioral therapy as the best method. The reality is that many techniques and schools of thought can be helpful. Many situations we find ourselves in are complicated; a good therapist can shed light on your specific issue and provide helpful insight. Moral support is also critical.

For some reason, many people are resistant to seeking psychotherapy. I am always perplexed as to why that would be the case. We all have experienced less than perfect modeling from our parents. I have yet to meet anyone from a perfectly "functional" family that has left them with no emotional baggage.

I think of life as a backpacking trip. Why would you go on the trip with fifty pounds of rocks in your pack in addition to basic supplies? Therapy helps you unload those useless rocks.

I would suggest that if you don't believe in therapy—or just plain don't want to go—you're choosing to remain a victim of your circumstances. I find it surprising that some patients in chronic pain who are under stress refuse to talk to a therapist but are eager to undergo an operation that carries significant risk. There really is no downside risk of talking to a therapist.

### Self-Help Books

There are tens of thousands of self-help books available. During one period of my life I was obsessive about reading one after another. I do feel that they can be a helpful and even necessary piece of working on oneself. They represent a didactic phase of learning about life skills and most of the authors are smart, experienced people.

Self-help books can be a good resource, but my counselor eventually ordered me to quit reading them. He saw the danger they posed, which is that they can become a substitute for actual change. I tended to intellectualize them and they became another part of my identity. Although I thought I'd made the correct changes, I hadn't gone into the experiential phase enough to have anything really take place; it was all conceptual. However, they did sow the seeds for real change.

### Structured Seminars

Attending structured seminars focused on self-discovery can be a good step toward finding your true self because they add an experiential level to the process. In addition, sharing what you're learning with others who are on the same quest is very powerful.

There are many seminars available. I don't have any specific recommendations; I think most of them have a lot of potential value if you commit to the process and can connect to it. If, by chance, you have negative feelings about a given seminar, it might be because you have different needs, or because you're not ready to deal with the issues it has raised, or maybe because seminars are simply not an effective resource for you. Just don't give up on the self-discovery process as a whole.

### The Quiet Mind

This quote from Bernie Siegel, author of *Love, Medicine, and Miracles* pretty well sums up the essence of the DOC project:

*The issue is the quiet mind*
*Then the truth can be seen*
*In mythology it is the still pond where the true image is reflected back*
*to you*
*And also when you can truly be in touch with your unconscious and*
*communicate*
*Through it with yourself and others*
*It is the reason we sleep also*
*To quiet the thinking mind and feel and see the truth*
*As an attorney said,*
*"While learning to think I almost forgot how to feel."*
Bernie Siegel, MD

I agree with Dr. Siegel that a quiet mind is a necessary requirement to move forward. Think of planning a ten-day vacation. You would either sit down in a calm, relatively quiet space and research it online; buy travel books or look at them at the library; or you might talk to a travel agent. You would not attempt to do this while attending a rock concert. Don't forget that, if you've been battling chronic mental and physical pain for a while, the noise in your head is probably very loud.

### Sitting Quietly

When I think of moving forward and taking action, I also think of the Native Americans. When hunting or moving camp they would send out scouts to assess the situation for opportunities and danger. Much of it was spent quietly watching. When they were tracking game they would use every visual and auditory cue and were incredibly quiet. They were not yelling at each other across the valley. When was the last time that you just sat quietly and carefully considered all of your options?

## Connecting with Others

Human consciousness evolved by humans interacting with other humans.[5] It is no coincidence that most of my patients suffering from chronic pain indicate on my intake questionnaire that they are isolated from others. I have observed a distinct interplay between anxiety, anger, pain, and social isolation. It might have something to do with the fact that anger is a self-centered, survival reaction that is far from attractive. Regardless of the reason, anger disconnects you from you, others, and your surroundings. It also binds you to the past. Using the approaches in this book, you can break this cycle. It cannot be done solely by intellectual methods.

As you disentangle yourself from your web of negativity, the next step is reconnecting with the world, beginning with your family and close friends. Many of my patients view this as a critical step in their healing. As a different part of your brain reawakens, and reward chemicals flood your body, you will think more clearly and just feel better overall, in spite of the pain.

As you connect with others you continue to move forward by seeing life from a larger perspective. Simply considering the possibilities beyond the human experience can be a spiritual practice, which you may choose to express in a religious manner; but that would be only a small part of your spiritual journey. Keeping an open mind is key.

As your perspective grows, you will move farther and farther away from your pain circuits; and as you use these negative pathways less, they will atrophy, allowing the more pleasurable ones to grow. Within this process lies the ultimate answer to your suffering

## Expanding Your Horizon—Final Thoughts

The essence of the DOC process is simply chilling out and moving on. You can't have one without the other. An equally crucial DOC principle is to move forward with your life, with or without your pain. If you are waiting for your pain to abate before you live your life, the pain is running the show. Paradoxically, the farther you move along in the process, the higher the chance your pain will decrease or disappear.

The final and most important thought is that there is no goal to the DOC program. People often become overwhelmed with all the exercises to do and books to read, expecting a long journey ahead of them. In reality, the "goal" of this journey is simply to connect whatever moment you are in with the tools you now possess, which will become easier over time.

But there is no endpoint. You can fully engage, right this second, by simply placing your attention on what is in front of you and becoming aware of your reaction.

Welcome to your new life.

# Appendix A: Do You Really Need Surgery?

Medicine has become big business—and you, the patient, are a hot commodity. You and your health problems are the main source of revenue for many companies that need to report hefty profits to their shareholders. In this era of so-called health reform, it's important to understand what this means to you, the patient—and the news is not good.

As a spine surgeon, I enjoy caring for patients. I perform surgeries when they are necessary and will help people feel better and function well. Unfortunately, many people getting spine surgery today not only won't be helped—they'll suffer more as a result of the unexpected consequences that result from surgeries they could have avoided.

For example, let's look at spinal fusion. There is clear research showing that only about 25 percent of patients significantly benefit from a spine fusion for lower back pain (LBP).[1] A report from Washington State, where I practice, showed that just 15 percent of people who've had spinal fusion have returned to work one year after their operation.[2]

Physicians today are trained to use evidence-based data to make treatment decisions—and yet when it comes to low back pain, the data is routinely ignored. A recent study showed that physicians eschew established clinical guidelines for best practices in treating back pain.[3] Patient risk factors for poor surgical outcomes include lack of sleep, anxiety, depression, catastrophizing (overreacting), and situational stresses. A 2014 paper reported that less than 10 percent of surgeons assess and consider these factors when making a surgical decision for their patients.[4]

A visiting neurosurgical resident once spent a week with me, watching how I deal with non-operative care. He told me that the only exposure he'd had in his training for non-operative care was to write "physical therapy" on a prescription pad and send the patient on their way. Yet by the day he graduates he will have the ability to determine if a patient has indeed "failed" conservative care.

## Surgical Nightmares

In my years in practice, I've run across many patients who have had terrible experiences with surgery. I've included them here to demonstrate the importance of approaching surgery with caution.

George was a middle-aged businessman with LBP. For his back pain, he had a spinal fusion that had a low chance of success. When it didn't help, he had another one. As a result of complications from the second surgery, he lost bowel and bladder function and now walks with crutches.

Teresa was an athletic young woman who was struck in the back by a swinging steel beam while at work. Although it was a significant blow, there were no fractures; she simply suffered a bruise to her spine. Despite this, she underwent fifteen sets of injections and then was fused from her neck to her pelvis. Unfortunately, she was fused incorrectly, leaving her unable to stand up. I had to spend another ten hours surgically cutting her spine in two and re-straightening her.

Tom was an older gentleman who was in poor physical condition.

He had spinal stenosis (constricted nerves) that was not severe enough to cause leg pain. He underwent a fusion from his tenth thoracic vertebrae to the pelvis and developed a deep wound infection. Then his spine broke down and pinched his spinal cord just above the steel rods at his ninth thoracic vertebra. He became partially paraplegic and had to be fused up to his neck. Fortunately, he regained the strength in his legs.

Amanda is a young woman who has undergone four fusions of her lower back in the last five years, and they still have not healed. I will have to spend eight hours redoing her surgery to make it solid.

I have hundreds of stories like this, and they all share one common theme. Each person had a normally aging spine before any surgery was done; none of them required any surgery—especially a fusion. Fusions are necessary and helpful only for unstable or deformed spines; they do not relieve back pain. Each patient would have done very well with a structured spine care program and limited treatment.

George, Teresa, and Tom all would have done well with physical therapy and a self-directed structured rehabilitation program. Amanda needed a more comprehensive program but surgery should not have been a choice, from my perspective. Her spine imaging studies prior to surgery were normal for her age.

Instead, all these patients have been subjected to unspeakable misery that has altered their lives. The costs to society from failed spine surgery in both dollars and human suffering are enormous.

Sarah is an older woman who came to me for a second opinion after she felt she was being rushed in to major deformity surgery to correct her leaning forward and to the right. In talking to her, I discovered she'd lost her daughter to drowning within the month before seeing the surgeon. No one who's grieving should have surgery. She may have eventually benefitted from surgery but she was not in a state of mind to make that decision.

### Why So Much Surgery?

Our surgical training is geared toward defining and dealing with the pain source. We are taught to think mechanically. There are many structural spine problems that can be solved or ameliorated with surgery, and there's nothing more rewarding than performing a technically excellent operation where the patient does well. But unfortunately, the mechanical solution mindset is also applied to low back pain, which does not usually come from a structural problem.

I am a surgeon who has been on both sides of this fence. I spent the first eight years of my practice aggressively offering fusion surgery to my lower back pain patients because I felt it was the correct choice. For a long time, I felt obligated to offer *something*. But gradually it dawned on me that fusion surgeries were hurting more than helping, and it took me a few years to learn to say, "No, I cannot surgically help you out." I finally stopped doing them around 1994. Only in looking back do I see how little I knew about the pain experience during the early years of my practice.

The pressure to do fusions comes from patients as well as doctors. When a patient sees a surgeon, it's often implied that everything else that can be done has been done. This visit represents the last resort. When I tell my patients, no, they sometimes explode in anger because they feel that I don't believe them and am refusing to solve their problem. The promise of a definitive procedure is the first thing on many patients' minds.

### The Business of Medicine

When it comes to back pain, the unpleasant physical symptoms you feel are more likely a result of the body's chemical response to your surroundings than a fixable structural problem. Healers figured this out centuries ago and often healed by calming people down. With the advent of technology in the early twentieth century, we have completely switched directions. If someone is having abdominal pain, physicians will immediately order a battery of tests, including an endoscopy, instead of finding out whether the patient is, for example, being verbally abused at home or bullied at school.

The major forces creating the current procedure-oriented state of affairs in the medical profession include:

- Lack of physician training about chronic pain.
- Super specialization—doctors tend to stay within their area of expertise.
- Financial incentives skewed heavily toward procedures instead of long-term health.
- Increasing number of physicians employed by the hospitals.
- Physicians routinely ignoring best clinical practices guidelines, as documented in multiple research papers.

You may have heard about the contribution of electronic medical records to patient safety. There is easier access to your medical records, communication between providers is enhanced, and medication errors are reduced. These are all significant factors that improve the safety and quality of your care.

These same computerized records are also used to monitor every keystroke that your physician enters into the medical record. This includes the number of diagnostic tests ordered and procedures performed. Physicians are then profiled by their "contribution to the profitability of the institution." The more procedures and tests that are done on you, the more value your doctor has to the institution and the more say they have on how medicine is practiced.

Not only are physicians not being financially rewarded for talking to their patients, they are being profiled in a negative fashion for not being aggressive in ordering tests and performing procedures. The problem with this practice is that, typically, most of the profitable procedures being prescribed *do not work*, while the less expensive, *effective* strategies are ignored!

Some additional factors to consider:

- Cortisone injections for back pain haven't been shown to be effective in any study, either in the short or long term. They can provide some mild temporary benefit for leg pain or sciatica.

- Facet injections are not only ineffective, they are not being done correctly. The procedure is supposed to be done at only one level with both a long-acting and short-acting local anesthetic at two different times. The pain relief, if present, should correlate with the duration of the anesthetic effect. Preferably, this should be repeated a couple of times before a *facet rhizotomy* is performed. This is a procedure where the small sensory nerves around the joints in the back of your spine are either burned or frozen. Relief can occur for up to a year if the above steps are followed. Most patients currently receive one set of multiple-level injections with one anesthetic, and the rhizotomies performed are based on very vague data. All of this is expensive and time-consuming. Some centers demand payment in cash to do all of this in one day.

- Physical therapy that uses only modalities such as heat, ice, and ultrasound can give some short-term relief. However, it's not nearly as effective as analyzing your body mechanics, tendon inflammation, range of motion of the surrounding joints; and then performing focused manual therapy.

- Many patients don't set up a long-term conditioning program, which is a vital part of rehabilitation, as they find it too time-consuming.

- Doctors hastily prescribe anti-depressants and anti-anxiety medications rather than finding out what may be actually going on with their patients. Once he or she prescribes medications, your physician feels that that part of your care is covered. Unfortunately, antidepressants don't work much better than a placebo. There might be a 10 percent improvement over a placebo, but that is not nearly effective as defined counseling. In a feature article in the *New York Times* a few years ago, a psychiatrist admitted to switching from psychotherapy to prescribing medications because it was much more lucrative, even though he knew that it was less effective.[5]

- The actual success rate of a spine fusion for LBP is less than 30 percent at two-year follow-up. One Ohio Worker's Compensation study showed that only 26 percent of employees who had the procedure returned to work within two years of surgery whereas that number was 67 percent in the non-surgical group. Twenty-seven percent had to undergo further surgery within the first year and 36 percent had complications.[6] There are still hundreds of thousands of these surgeries being performed every year. A significant part of my practice constitutes trying to salvage the damage done by aggressive surgeries that never needed to be done.

- Do patients really know what the success rate of a spine fusion is, versus the risks? When I gave a lecture in Phoenix to a spine business summit, I asked the group how many of them would consider a fusion for low back pain if the success rate were 50 percent (which is higher than the actual rate). No one raised their hand.

- There are very few surgeons I know that would undergo the same fusion surgery that they are recommending for their patients.

The bottom line is that overall, the explosion of technology has worsened, not improved, the level of health care. Technology precipitated the shift to performing a rapidly increasing number of procedures; this trend has been accelerated by medicine becoming a business.

## "Prehab"

The vast majority of my patients never require surgery. When it *is* necessary, outcomes can be significantly improved by using the DOC principles to address all of the variables that affect the perception of pain. I made up the name, "prehab," as I was developing a rehabilitation program for my patients to do before surgery. Based on the medical literature over the last thirty years, I have instituted the following protocol for all of my elective spine surgeries.

First and foremost, surgery is only a possibility if there is an identifiable structural problem with matching symptoms. Otherwise, it is off the table. If the patient improves enough during prehab, surgery is not done. This is the case with structural as well as nonstructural issues.

I want my patients to engage in the treatment plan for at least eight weeks prior to making the final decision regarding surgery, but there is no limit as to how long the treatment plan may last. The more a person immerses themselves in these concepts, the higher the chance of a successful outcome. If a patient doesn't want to engage in the program, then I will decline to be their surgeon.

Here is a rough outline of my expectations. It is not a formal program.

1. You are consistently getting a restful night's sleep.
2. You are using stress management tools and have seen some improvement in anxiety and frustration levels.
3. An exercise program is in place, which may or may not include physical therapy.
4. Medications have been defined and stabilized, especially long-term narcotic use.

5. You have a basic understanding about the complexity of chronic pain, including neurophysiologic disorder (NPD).

6. Specific goals are set from the beginning of treatment, not just, "I want to get rid of my pain" or "I want my life back."

There's an understanding of the specific goals of the proposed operative procedure. Spine surgery will not reliably relieve neck pain, thoracic pain, or LBP. Frequently, patients will cancel surgery when they realize it's only intended to relieve leg or arm symptoms.

Remember that you are the only one who can assess whether the severity of your pain is bad enough to take on the risks of surgery—including making the pain much worse. You are the one who has to take responsibility for the criteria being met. A surgeon cannot get inside your head. We base our decisions on our own filters and what you are saying. Learn what's at stake instead of relying on anyone else to present this information. This is a higher stakes game than you might think.

## Never Should Have Had Surgery

A few years ago, I took care of Jeff, a psychologist in his mid-thirties, who'd spontaneously developed episodic low back pain about ten years earlier. The pain would occur two to three times a year and last approximately seven to ten days. Between these episodes he was symptom-free, and his lifestyle wasn't limited by pain.

After several years of on-and-off pain, Jeff went to see a surgeon and was told that he had degenerated discs and would benefit from a spine fusion. Minimal rehabilitation had been tried. He went ahead with the fusion, which did not heal. He then experienced more severe pain and had a second operation to repair the fusion. Although it was successfully repaired, his pain still did not diminish. He came to me because a "new procedure" had been proposed: inserting flexible rods above the fusion, across the next disc space.

By this time, Jeff was almost housebound with unrelenting pain, and on methadone. Methadone is a strong, long-acting narcotic, which merely took the edge off of his pain. He was still in some pain and also groggy from the narcotics. He continued to work as a psychologist part-time, but his overall quality of life was poor.

My recommendation was not to undergo further surgery. Jeff's situation was a tragedy in that, based on our conversation, I could tell that he hadn't had enough pain in the first place to warrant surgery. It's tricky in that the surgeon had probably heard him say "five years of pain," and felt surgery was a reasonable option. The patient heard that his back could be made better. He didn't comprehend the possibility that surgical intervention might make his situation much worse. I never heard back from Jeff after his appointment and I'm guessing he had yet another failed procedure.

Unfortunately, Jeff's situation is common and a significant part of my practice. I am the "salvage surgeon." Being educated enough to make a truly informed decision is critical. Surgeries are elective, and you—only you—should make the final call.

## Flawed Studies

There have been many studies done on fusions for LBP, but most of them share a major flaw: a high percentage of the subjects didn't participate in study follow-up and/or could not be located at the two-year post-surgery point that is the standard follow-up time for most clinical research projects. One has to assume that patients lost to follow-up are doing poorly. We know that patients who have poor outcomes are generally upset and less likely to volunteer their time years later. You also cannot assume a good result when the result is not known. Taking that into account, marginal results become unacceptable. Often problems come up after the two-year mark, such as a breakdown of the spine around the fusion, non-healing of the fusion, and failure of the hardware. One Washington

State study revealed an overall re-operation rate of 19 percent for all spine surgeries.[7] Another glitch: most studies define a successful outcome as a 25 percent improvement for pain and function. My bet is that if you are getting a spinal fusion, you're expecting to become pain-free, not just 25 percent better. Lastly, none of the studies compared surgery to carefully planned structured rehab.

Dr. Peter Fritzell's research paper[8] is the one I hear most often quoted in support of using fusion for degenerated discs in the lower back. The study was funded by a spinal implant manufacturer.

In the study, there were 222 patients in the surgical group and 72 in the non-surgical group. (The surgical group was larger because they were using the study to compare three different types of surgical procedures.) When I reviewed the information, I noticed a problem right away. Not enough care was taken in the diagnosis phase. In the study, the decision to perform a fusion was made in part by feel: the surgeon pushed on each patient's spine to find the specific spinal segment that produced a painful response. However, no X-rays were taken during this pushing maneuver to confirm and document the surgeon's findings. An X-ray is critical in preventing the most common complication in spine surgery: operating on the wrong segment. Making the decision to do such a large surgical intervention (the fusion) without X-ray confirmation is, in my mind, highly questionable. There is also no evidence suggesting that pushing on the spine is a valid diagnostic test.

In the surgical group, there was a fairly impressive decrease in pain during the initial six months after surgery. However, at the two-year follow-up, the pain had significantly increased. The final overall reduction in pain was about 30 percent. The improvement in function was 25 percent. Depression decreased about 20 percent.

The patients in the surgical group had about double the improvement in almost all parameters compared to the non-surgical group.

Based on these results, researchers concluded that the data supported the use of a fusion for low back pain. I question the results, however— the statistics are skewed because of the non-treatment for the nonoperative group. As we've established, random treatments for chronic pain are simply not effective in the long-term. I am surprised that the non-surgical group had any improvement at all, as untreated chronic pain usually worsens with time.

One interesting note: the study's overall complication rate of 24 percent (50 out of 211 surgeries) reveals the serious risks of surgery. The major complications noted included deep wound infection, blood clots, and pneumonia. Eight percent (16 out of 211) required an additional unintended trip back to the operating room. Surgery should not be taken lightly.

### Worth the Risk?

One of my concerns about patients who are considering surgery for low back pain is that they haven't been given a full picture of the risks involved. When a patient is offered a spinal fusion, it's typically implied to them that there's a 70 to 80 percent chance of success. In other words, they're told it's likely they'll emerge almost pain-free. However, there's little consistent evidence to support that success rate.

Even if the success rate were 70 percent, would surgery be worth the risk? Many patients say yes—they're in so much pain they feel they can't turn it down. They desperately want to think it will work. In my experience, though, most patients and many surgeons don't really comprehend how bad the aftermath of a failed spine surgery can be. This is one of the main reasons that I have written this book.

I've had a few patients say that even if the success rate is only 10 percent, they still want the operation. If I reverse that, though, and point out that the chance of failure is 90 percent, they think about it a little differently.

If surgery doesn't go well, it can lead to more procedures and more pain. If none of the subsequent procedures work, it can be disastrous. The "disaster factor" has to be fully understood before making the decision to undergo a fusion.

## A Careful Study

The study that firmly confirmed my observations on fusions for LBP was directed by Eugene Carragee, an orthopedic spine surgeon at Stanford Hospital in Palo Alto, CA.[1] In a small but meticulous study, Dr. Carragee argued that if a test called the discogram was a valid test for back pain caused by degenerated discs (non-structural pain), then the "gold standard" reason for performing a spine fusion, the fusion should predictably result in pain relief for this condition. He took a degenerated disc group and compared it to a group who had gross instability in their backs.

To review, a discogram is a test where dye is injected directly into your disc and a physician observes your pain response. If the response is similar to your usual pain, a fusion or artificial disc is considered.

The issue I have with the discogram is that it's a subjective test: it depends on both the patient's and physician's interpretations of pain, and there is also a lot of variation in technique. It has also been shown that patients under stress are more sensitive to pain and are therefore more likely to experience pain from the injection. Therefore, I don't consider it reliable for making a structural diagnosis.

Dr. Carragee had the discograms for the degenerated disc group performed in a very careful manner, with every detail documented. In addition, detailed psychological tests revealed that none of the thirty-two patients had significant outside life stresses.

The group with instability, consisting of thirty-four patients, had a structural issue in the form of a bone defect called a "pars defect." Each person had at least 4 mm of abnormal motion when they bent forward and backwards under an X-ray. In our spine surgical world, this is quite a significant insta-bility. It's believed that a fusion in this situation will work the vast majority of the time. This group, like the first, was documented to have no notable life stresses.

The surgical result for the bony defect group was a 72 percent satisfactory outcome. In the non-structural discogram group, the surgical success rate was 27 percent. One hundred percent of the patients participated in follow-up.

It was surprising to me that the structural group had only a 72 percent success rate; I would have expected well over 90 percent. That tells me that even with a structural problem, there is a significant soft tissue component. And what about the possibility of NPD?

The low success rate in the discogram/degenerated disc group was surprising as well. Under the circumstances, I would have estimated it would to be close to 50 percent. Carragee's attention to detail on the quality of discography was extremely high; additionally, he had done his best to screen out patients who were under a lot of stress. Nevertheless, 27 percent doesn't even approach the placebo response.

These tests were performed on patients with low stress. Given the results, do you think it's likely that a fusion could relieve LBP in someone who has been off of work for three years and is frustrated beyond words? The answer is probably not. A recent paper shows that even if you have a well-done, warranted operation in the face of chronic pain, there is a significant chance that your pain will be made worse. Pre-operative chronic pain is a major predictor of experiencing post-op-erative chronic pain.[9]

Although Carragee's study is a small one, no other study has been conducted with nearly his amount of precision and follow-up. If a study emerges that is larger and as well done, I will look at it. If it comes to the opposite conclusion, I will reconsider my whole approach to surgery for LBP. However, today that study does not exist. The studies that suggest surgery is warranted for LBP are seriously flawed, not only because they don't follow patients for more than two years, but also because of poor screening, low percentage of patients followed-up on, vague selection criteria, and over-enthusiastic interpretation of the results. The data is misleading to surgeons in training. Be very careful about your decision to have surgery for back pain based on degenerative disc disease. It does not work often enough to warrant the risks.

## Twenty-Nine Surgeries

Doug was a twenty-five-year-old steel worker who ruptured a disc in his lower back, which caused sciatica. He had a discectomy (disc removal) for the sciatica but was still experiencing low back pain so severe that he couldn't return to work. His doctors couldn't locate the source of his pain, so I would consider it non-structural. After two years of physical therapy, he was still in pain and extremely frustrated, understandably. He elected to undergo a fusion.

This first fusion was the start of a long and painful two decades for Doug. There were so many complications that by the time he saw me at age forty-eight, he'd undergone nineteen operations and was on high-dose narcotics. His fusion now extended from his neck to his pelvis. He'd never returned to work.

I was able to perform a series of operations that restored Doug's posture and greatly improved his quality of life. The improvement lasted for only about a year, though. A serious wound infection occurred, which required that his spinal screws and rods be removed, and his spine bent forward again.

The cycle continued, and recently Doug had two more major operations. The procedures re-straightened his spine initially, but three weeks later, he again developed a serious deep wound infection that required surgical drainage. He is now up to twenty-nine surgeries and counting. He has done pretty well for the last couple of years and we are both encouraged. But how much of the prime of his life has been consumed by failed spine surgeries?

The tragedy with Doug is that the fusion that started all his problems was likely unnecessary. Chances are that his extreme frustration sensitized his nervous system and led to much of his initial pain. Almost every patient I see who has undergone multiple failed back surgeries had the original surgery to reduce pain with no identifiable source, much like Doug's low back pain (and Jeff's, above). When a major invasive procedure is done for a vague diagnosis, the potential downside can far outweigh the benefit. Even one unnecessary surgery can set you on a path that changes your life irrevocably.

## Putting Myself Out of Business

The biggest surprise of this project over the last two years has been that I have seen over fifty patients with severe structural problems cancel their surgery because their symptoms resolved during the prehab process. In the first edition of this book, I recommended undergoing surgery more aggressively if you had a structural problem in the face of chronic pain. My reasoning was that you could not tolerate the stress of additional pain. It has not worked out that way. It turns out that performing surgery in the presence of a fired-up nervous system is a bad idea regardless of whether you have a structural problem. Many patients will be made worse by surgery.

My realization was supported by several research papers I found documenting that a patient could have worse pain after any surgery up to 40 percent of the time in the presence of pre-existing chronic pain.[9] The prehab program was designed to avoid this scenario and also to improve the outcome of surgery. I never imagined that the pain would disappear without the surgery when the pathology was so severe. I now regularly see patients who feel better and cancel surgery. Even if they eventually elect to undergo an operation, the results have been much better. I have reached a phase in my practice where it has become almost impossible to sustain my work as a surgeon.

## A Final Word

Part of the tragedy of chronic pain is that once you have a failed back surgery, it's harder to get help. The surgeons who performed the surgery are not trained or comfortable in dealing with chronic pain. Other surgeons are reluctant to get involved in managing another surgeon's failures. The non-surgeons do the best they can to improve your quality of life, but they often take on a survival mentality for chronic pain patients, not a proactive one.

Many patients become extremely upset if they're told that they aren't good candidates for surgery. They feel like their last hope has been taken away. I understand the frustration. It's as if you've finally reached the mountaintop and discovered you were climbing the wrong mountain.

If you're told you *are* a good candidate, I know that it's hard not to take your surgeon up on the offer. Pain puts you in a vulnerable position. You do want to believe in surgery.

It's much better, though, to develop your own resources for recovery instead of looking to surgery as the only answer. You'll be more open to employing these resources once you understand all the factors that brought you down into the Abyss. The DOC program evolved from my own struggle with chronic pain as well as my observations of what has helped my patients regain control of their lives. I am continually inspired by their determination and successes.

# Appendix B: Self-Inventory Template

**Overview of Self Today:**

Core Values

- Self
- Family
- Friends
- Career
- Financial
- Giving back

Character

- Strengths
- Flaws

Skills

- Highest (expert)
- Strong (competent and can contribute)
- Moderate (competent)
- Light (participant)

Dreams

**Where Do I Want to Be in Five Years?**

- Overview
- Specific areas
  - Self
  - Family
  - Friends
  - Career
  - Financial
  - Giving back

**Action Plan for This Year**

- Each area
  - Specific steps
  - Time frames

# Acknowledgments

I AM INCREDIBLY GRATEFUL TO BE ABLE TO SHARE with you the knowledge I gained through surviving a severe burnout. It included intense chronic emotional and physical pain. I would not have made it through without the support of my wife, Babs. It can most simply be said that she was able to see the best in me. When we met in 2001 I was careening into the Abyss. How she was able to ride out this phase of my life with me is a mystery.

My colleagues around Seattle have been very supportive of my efforts and I have appreciated their clear feedback and exchange of ideas. They include David Tauben, Stan Herring, Stu Weinstein, Gordon Irving, David Cassius, Joel Konikow, and Jim Robinson.

Stuart Eivers and Mark Trombold are two excellent physical therapists who reviewed Chapter 16 on rehabilitation. I appreciate their expert opinion on a broad topic.

Howard Schubiner, M.D. is a pain specialist from Detroit, Michigan, who was one of the keynote speakers at a seminar, "A Course on Compassion: Empathy in the Face of Chronic Pain." He taught me that what I was inadvertently treating was the mind-body syndrome and what I call neurophysiologic disorder. His concepts are expressed throughout the book.

My son Nick and his best friend Holt Haga, who are both world-class freestyle mogul skiers, have been inspirational in teaching me to deal with adversity. They have also supplied ample material for many of the stories in this book.

Tom Masters and Mark Mendonca have been part of the core team making every aspect of this book possible. I have appreciated their talent and commitment to getting these concepts into the world.

Ray Bunnage, a good friend and creative computer programmer, has spent hundreds of hours looking at the literature supporting the concepts. His efforts have provided a profound depth of knowledge to this book. Our discussions have stimulated many new ideas.

David Elaimy, my golf instructor and surgical performance coach, has remarkable insights into the stresses we experience under competitive conditions. I have been able to apply his wisdom to the rest of my life. Many of my ideas are a result of our extensive conversations.

My stepdaughter, Jaz, has truly been an inspiration. She has come through her teenage years with flying colors while experiencing her own set of stresses. She has been also very clear in her feedback about the principles outlined in this book.

It was also through Jaz that our family was introduced to the Hyde School, which was founded by Joey Gauld. Hyde is based on the concept that character development is the most important focus of education. Joey has been a remarkable inspiration and showed me that it is important to follow the path of who you truly are.

At the age of eighty, Joey Gauld went through the Hoffman Process during Jaz's senior year. As a result, my wife, my son, daughter-in-law, and I also went through it. I was not prepared for any of the changes that occurred during those eight days. A special thanks to my Hoffman teachers, Kani Comstock, Barbara Comstock, and Raz Ingrazci. Through them, I learned that I cannot change anyone except myself.

Marty and Marilyn Chattman have opened their home in the Dominican Republic to Babs and me. Over half of this book was written during the weeks down there when I was able to get truly relaxed. Thank you!

Anne Cole Norman has been editing this book from the beginning and has been instrumental in developing the message. Thank you to Lisa Carlson and the Cadence Group, who worked on the copy editing. I also greatly appreciated Marilyn Alan, who meticulously did the final edits. Alfio Cini is a dear friend in Italy who is a talented art director. He is responsible for the cover design.

Finally, I want to thank my patients who have inspired me with their determination to get their lives back. Given the slightest chance, they have fought through indescribable circumstances back to health. This is the fuel that pushes me forward. I am grateful that I have been able to be the catalyst that has started the healing process.

# GLOSSARY

**Acute**—Sudden onset, severe; requiring immediate attention.

**ANTS**—Automatic negative thoughts—Term used by David Burns in his book, *Feeling Good,* which describes the mind's tendency to gravitate toward negative thoughts.

**Adrenaline**—A "fight or flight" hormone secreted by the adrenal glands in response to a real or perceived threat. Effects include an increased heart rate, sweating, rapid breathing, muscle tension, and feeling agitated.

**Affective component**—The emotional component of pain as opposed to the somatosensory aspect (see below).

**Anxiety**—The feeling that is generated by the body's stress hormones such as adrenaline and cortisol.

**Anxiolytics**—Category of medications that directly decrease anxiety.

**Axial**—Refers to the center of the body excluding the arms and legs.

**Bibliotherapy**—Applying any type of therapy just through the use of a book.

**C-reactive protein (CRP)**—A chemical marker that signals inflammation in the body. Can be elevated in infection, autoimmune disorders, and stress.

**Central sensitization syndrome (CSS)**—A term indicating the nervous system is more sensitive to stress. The conduction velocity of the nerves increases.

**Chondromalacia patella**—Pain under the kneecap associated with softening of the cartilage between the patella and the end of the femur. It is especially sensitive when going up and down stairs.

**Chronic pain**—The classic definition is "pain that lasts longer than the expected healing time." With recent advances in neuroscience research it has been redefined as "a maladaptive neuropathological disease state" that creates symptoms that are not consistent with the injury or environment.

**Cognitive behavioral therapy (CBT)**—The branch of psychology that specifically addresses dysfunctional belief systems along with the associated behaviors.

**Cognitive distortions**—Thought patterns or belief systems that are not consistent with reality.

**Congenital indifference to pain**—A disorder where babies are born without a protective pain system. Since they usually cannot protect themselves, they become quickly disfigured and live less than twenty years.

**Cortisol**—The body's stress hormone that regulates metabolism and the immune system. Adrenaline and cortisol are considered the two main hormones that regulate the body's ability to fend off internal and external threats to survival.

**Diabetic mono-neuritis**—Elevated blood sugars can cause hypersensitivity and severe pain in the pathway of a nerve. It is important that this condition not be misdiagnosed as a pinched nerve.

**Dissociating**—In the context of mental processes, it is the act of consciously or unconsciously separating from the past. This an extreme form of thought suppression.

**Discogram**—A procedure where an iodine dye is injected into a lumbar disc in an attempt to reproduce a patient's low back pain.

**DOC (define your own care) process**—A self-directed program consisting of strategies to take control of your own treatment of chronic pain.

**Endorphins/enkephalins**—These are the body's natural pain killers and are many times stronger than narcotics. They are secreted in response to pain and are a part of the body's stress response.

**Expressive writing**—Several hundred research papers have documented that simply writing down positive or negative thoughts and feelings on paper has a dramatic effect on physical symptoms, performance, and mood. It is necessary to immediately destroy the paper so you can write with absolute freedom and avoid analyzing what you wrote.

**Facets**—Two small joints in the back of each level of the spine. They have the same structure as all other articular joints (have cartilage and are contained by a capsule of connective tissue). There is ongoing debate regarding their role in generating back pain.

**Facet rhizotomy**—The facet joint capsules have an abundant number of pain fibers. There is debate about whether these sensory nerves are potentially a source of pain. A rhizotomy utilizes heat or cold to destroy these small sensory fibers and if the joint capsule is the source of pain, then LBP will be decreased. The pain fibers grow back within about a year.

**Failed back syndrome**—Refers to patients who have undergone multiple failed back surgeries. One of the main reasons I am writing this book is to prevent this tragedy from happening to you. The downside of a failed spine surgery can be catastrophic.

**Fascia**—Envelopes of tissue surrounding muscles that contain and define them. There is an abundant number of pain receptors in this layer.

**Flatback**—Loss of the curvature of the lower back can occur as the result of surgery or as part of the aging process. As the lordosis decreases, it causes your head to hang forward in relationship to the pelvis. Flatback refers to the decreased lordosis in the lumbar spine.

**Functional MRI (fMRI)**—By injecting a labeled glucose (this sugar is the brain's energy source), MRI scans can pick up which parts of the brain are active in relationship to specific activities and emotions.

**Hip arthritis—degenerative**—Arthritis refers to the destruction of the cartilage of a joint. Cartilage traps water and provides a cushion between bones that allows joints to move. Degenerative arthritis occurs when this cushion wears out and eventually there is only bone against bone. Interestingly, there is no correlation between the severity of arthritis in the spine, hip, knee, or shoulder and the intensity of pain.

**Hippocampus**—An area of the brain that is responsible for processing long- and short-term memory.

**Hoffman Process**—In the 1960s, Robert Hoffman founded a process that has evolved into a seven-day workshop. It's a remarkably effective program that creates an awareness of one's family patterns, allows you to separate from them, and then reprogram. This book would never have been written without the Hoffman Process workshop I attended in 2009. I still use the tools daily.

**Iliotibial band (IT)**—A wide tendon that connects the pelvis to the lower leg and stabilizes your leg as you walk.

**"Ironic effect"**—Dr. Daniel Wegner introduced this term from the results of his research on suppressing negative thoughts. The "ironic effect" describes the process of thinking about something more when you try not to think about it; and thinking about it less if you try to think about it.

**Junction box**—My term for the sum total of all the nervous system's activity at a given moment.

**Laminectomy**—The back part of the spinal canal is protected by a bone that is called the lamina. To surgically address the pathology within the spinal canal it is necessary to remove this bone. A complete removal of the lamina is a laminectomy, whereas a partial removal is a laminotomy.

**Leaning into the negative**—A term coined by Gabriele Oettingen in her book, *Rethinking Positive Thinking,* which means allowing yourself to experience your negative feelings. It is important to become aware of your automatic survival responses before you can substitute more functional ones.

**Lordosis**—One of the functions of the spine is to keep your head balanced over your pelvis. There is a curvature both in the neck and lower back that accomplishes this and the curvature is referred to as lordosis. The thoracic spine has curvature that is the reverse of the neck and lower back and is termed, "kyphosis."

**Maladaptive neuropathological disease state**—In chronic pain, the brain rewires in a way that is disconnected to actual sensory input. It is a maladaptive rewiring. With time, these circuits become permanent and create a disease state that manifests as any number of physical symptoms.

**Masking**—Covering up or avoiding.

**Mind-body syndrome (MBS)**—See "NPD."

**Myelin**—A fatty substance that surrounds nerve cells and improves conduction of impulses, similar to what insulation does for an electric wire.

**Muscle memory**—Muscles, actually, do not have memory. Muscle memory is neurological memory where repeatable pathways are memorized by the central nervous system. It is unclear how they are formed but myelin is a substance that "insulates" the pathways similar to the insulation on an electrical wire.

**Negative love syndrome**—This a Hoffman Process term that describes our need to adopt our parents' behavioral patterns in order to be accepted by our parents. My version of the process is simpler in that I think we just download environmental input. Unfortunately, most of our parents' coping patterns are normal human survival responses that are not helpful in creating an enjoyable life.

**Neural pathways**—Describes the repeatable circuits that are imbedded into our nervous system.

**Neuroplasticity**—The brain's capacity to adapt and change at any age.

**Neurological**—Descriptive term for anything to do with the nervous system.

**Neurophysiologic disorder (NPD)**—When you are exposed to chronic stress your body experiences prolonged elevation of the stress hormones, adrenaline and cortisol. As your body responds to these hormones, the result is a myriad of unpleasant symptoms. Chapter 2 lists over thirty different symptoms of NPD. Fortunately, as these hormones normalize, the symptoms resolve. Other terms for this disorder include:

- Mind-body syndrome (MBS)
- Psychophysiological disorder (PPD)
- Stress illness syndrome
- Psychosomatic disorder
- Tension myositis syndrome (TMS)

**Non-specific complaint**—In medicine, the reporting of vague physical symptoms. They can still represent a significant physical problem but are more difficult to sort out.

**Non-structural pain**—Pain that arises from irritation or inflammation of the soft tissues but has no identifiable anatomical abnormality.

**Obsessive-compulsive disorder (OCD)**—An anxiety disorder manifested by repetitive, intrusive thoughts. The thoughts usually fall into one of four categories: cleanliness, sexuality, violence, and religion. The response can be internal, with counter-thoughts; or external, with compulsive repetitive behaviors such as hand-washing.

**Over-adrenalized nervous system**—This is the state of your body when your body is exposed to sustained levels of adrenaline. Each organ of the body has a specific response.

**Pain generator**—Physicians, especially surgeons, are focused on finding a specific anatomic abnormality that is the cause of pain. However, it is much more likely that your body's symptoms are generated by the chemical response to sensory input from the environment.

**Peripheral nervous system**—This refers to any part of the nervous system that is distal to the brain or spinal cord. It transmits input from the environment to the central nervous system.

**Periosteum**—The layer of tissue covering bones. It is loaded with pain fibers and provides important feedback to the nervous system to protect the bones. It's also the reason that pain is so severe at the points where tendons and ligaments attach to bones.

**Phantom brain pain**—A term I have coined for disruptive obsessive thought patterns. Humans develop belief systems that are not connected to the reality in front of them and project their thoughts onto other people and situations. These spinning circuits are not responsive to rational conversation.

**Phantom limb pain**—Almost all amputees have experience of the limb still being there, and over half experience the pre-amputation pain.

**Physiology**—The function of living organisms.

**Pit of despair**—A cage used in Harry Harlow's lab, where he performed extensive research with primates regarding bonding. The cage was smaller at the bottom and the top was covered by a grate. The monkeys would climb up, look out, and slide back down. The monkeys would become depressed within a couple of days. His lab team was so upset by the experiment and called it "the pit of despair."

**Prehab**—A program requiring patients to engage in the DOC process for eight to twelve weeks prior to having elective surgery.

**Projection**—The process of attributing certain characteristics to another person when those thoughts really represent your interpretation of that person. Most of our opinions are simply our view of ourselves projected onto the world. This phenomenon completely clouds awareness.

**Psychological reflex**—When you're re-exposed to a similar situation that created a strong emotional response, your body will automatically respond in an identical manner.

**Psychophysiological disorder (PPD)**—See neurophysiologic disorder.

**Psychosomatic disorder**—See neurophysiologic disorder.

**REM sleep (Stage V)**—There are five stages of sleep. REM stands for "rapid eye movement" and it is the dreaming stage of sleep.

**Reflex sympathetic dystrophy (RSD)**—The pain that results from the autonomic nervous system being out of balance. The pain is often severe and unrelenting, with swelling and discoloration of the limb. It is unclear what sets off an imbalance. This part of the nervous system coordinates the involuntary control of your body and innervates smooth muscles, blood vessels, and other nerves. Its functions include dilating and constricting blood vessels.

**Reprogramming**—Learning any skill involves repetition before it becomes permanently imbedded in the nervous system. Reprogramming is the process of creating alternate pathways to a given stimulus.

**Scoliosis**—Sideways curvature of the spine.

**Somatosensory component**—Pain has both an emotional (affective) and physical component. The part of the nervous system that localizes the physical sensation to the body part is called the somatosensory component.

**Stress illness syndrome**—See neurophysiologic disorder.

**Subacute**—Acute pain that persists past the acute phase of several minutes, hours, or days. Pain lasting less than two months is considered subacute.

**Suppressing**—In the context of the DOC project, this is the conscious choice to avoid thinking and feeling unpleasant thoughts and emotions.

**Tennis elbow (lateral epicondylitis)**—Tendonitis on the outside of the elbow, from the origin of the tendons to your hands. The area becomes inflamed and painful, and it hurts to grip or engage in any activity that places tension on this area.

**Tension myositis syndrome (TMS)**—See neurophysiologic disorder.

**Triggering**—The nervous system's response to being exposed to situations that are similar to prior traumas.

**Unconstructive repetitive thoughts (URTs)**—Unpleasant thoughts that become more intrusive the more we attempt to control them.

**White bears experiment**—A nickname for the experiment designed by Dr. Daniel Wegner regarding thought suppression, where he asked his volunteers not to think about white bears.

# References

**Introduction**

1. Burns, David. *Feeling Good.* Avon Books, 1999.
2. Schubiner, Howard, and Michael Betzold. *Unlearn Your Pain.* Mind Body Publishing, 2010.
3. Luskin, Fred. *Forgive for Good.* Harper One, 2003.

**Chapter 1**

1. Davis KD and M Moayedi. "Central mechanisms of pain revealed through functional and structural MRI." *Journal of Neuroimmune Pharmacology* (2013); 8: 518–534.
2. Baliki MN and A Vania Apkarian. "Nociception, pain, negative moods, and behavior selection." *Neuron* (2015); 87: 474-491.
3. Tracey I and MC Bushnell. "How neuroimaging studies have challenged us to rethink: Is chronic pain a disease?" *The Journal of Pain* (2009); 10, 1113–1120.
4. Eisenberger N, et al. "Does rejection hurt? An fMRI study of social exclusion." *Science* (2003); 290.
5. Eisenberger N. "The neural bases of social pain: Evidence for shared representations with physical pain." *Psychosomatic Medicine* (2012); 74: 126-135.
6. Woo CW, et al. "Separate neural representations of physical pain and social rejection." *Nature Communications* (2014); DOI: 10.1038.
7. Wegener DM, et al. "Paradoxical effects of thought suppression." *Journal of Personality and Social Psychology* (1987); 53: 5-13.
8. Rahe R, et al. "Social stress and illness onset." *Journal of Psychosomatic Research* (1964); 8: 35.
9. Simons L, et al. "Pediatric Pain Screening Tool: rapid identification of risk in youth with pain complaints." *Pain* (2015); 156: 1511-1518.
10. Abbass A, et al. "Direct diagnosis and management of emotional factors in chronic headache patients." *Cephalgia* (2008); 28: 1305-1314.
11. Ballantyne J, et al. "Chronic pain after surgery or injury." *Pain: Clinical Updates - IASP* (2011); 19: 1-5.
12. Chen X, et al. "Stress enhances muscle nociceptor activity in the rat." *Neuroscience* (2011); 185: 166-173.

13. Evans, Patricia. *Verbal Abuse: Survivors Speak Out*. Avon Media Corporation, 1993.

14. Anda RF, et al. "The enduring effects of abuse and related adverse experiences in childhood. A convergence of evidence from neurobiology and epidemiology." *European Archives of Psychiatry and Clinical Neuroscience* (2006); 256: 174–186.

15. Copeland W, et al." Childhood bullying involvement predicts low-grade systemic inflammation into adulthood." *Proceedings of the National Academy of Science* (2014); 111: 7570-7575.

16. Trost Z, et al. "Cognitive dimensions of anger in chronic pain." *Pain* (2012); 153: 515-517.

## Chapter 2

1. Yancey, Philip, and Paul Brand. *Pain: The Gift Nobody Wants*. DIANE Publishing Company, 1999.

2. Schubiner, Howard, and Eric Keller. *Unlearn Your Pain*, 3rd edition. Mind Body Publishing, 2016.

3. Boden SD, et al. "Abnormal magnetic-resonance scans of the lumbar spine in asymptomatic subjects. A prospective investigation." *The Journal of Bone & Joint Surgery* (1990); 72:403– 8.

4. Nachemson A. "Advances in low back pain." *Clinical Orthopedics and Clinical Research* (1985); 200: 266-278.

5. Weinstein JN, et al. "Long-term follow-up of non-operatively treated thoracolumbar spine fractures." *Journal of Orthopedic Trauma* (1987); 1: 152-159.

6. Carragee EJ, et al. "A gold standard evaluation of the 'discogenic pain' diagnosis as determined by provocative discography." *Spine* (2006); 31: 2115-2123.

7. Lipton, Bruce. *Conversation in Santa Cruz*, CA, 2015.

8. Sarno, John. *Mind Over Back Pain*. Berkley Books, 1999.

## Chapter 3

1. Kahneman, Daniel. *Thinking Fast and Slow*. Farrar, Straus and Giroux, 2011.

2. Giesecke T, et al. "Evidence of augmented central pain processing in idiopathic chronic low back pain." *Arthritis and Rheumatism* (2004); 50: 613-623.

3. Hashmi, JA, et al. "Shape shifting pain: chronification of back pain shifts brain representation from nociceptive to emotional circuits." *Brain* (2013); 136: 2751–2768

4. Gallagher P, et al. "Phantom Limb Pain and RLP." *Disability and Rehabilitation* (2001); 23: 522-530.

5. Coyle, Daniel. *The Talent Code*. Bantam, 2009.

6. Ferrari R and D Louw. "Effect of a pain diary use on recovery from acute whiplash injury: a cohort study." *Journal of biomedicine & biotechnology* (2013); 14: 1049-1053.

7. Duruisseau S. and K. Schunke. *Medical Board of California Newsletter* (2007); 104: 1, 11, 17.

8. Schernhammer E. *New England Journal of Medicine* (2005); 352: 2473-2476.

9. Schernhammer E. *American Journal of Psychiatry* (2004); 161: 2295-2302.

10. Wegener DM, et al. "Paradoxical effects of thought suppression." *Journal of Personality and Social Psychology* (1987); 53: 5-13.

11. Garland E, et al. "Thought suppression as a mediator of the association between depressed mood and prescription opioid craving among chronic pain patients." *Journal of Behavavioral Medicine* (2016); 39: 128–138.

12. Hulbert J, et al. "Inducing amnesia through systemic suppression." *Nature Communications* (2016); 7: 1-9.

13. Seminowicz DA, et al. "Effective treatment of chronic low back pain in humans reverses abnormal brain anatomy and function." *The Journal of Neuroscience* (2011); 31: 7540-7550.

14. Oettengen, Gabriele. *Rethinking Positive Thinking: Inside the New Science of Motivation.* Current, 2014.

## Chapter 4

1. Chen X, et al. "Stress enhances muscle nociceptor activity in the rat." *Neuroscience* (2011); 185: 166-173.

2. Hossain J, et al. "The prevalence, cost implications, and management of sleep disorders: an overview." *Sleep and Breathing* (2002); 6: 85-102.

3. Karaman S, et al. "Prevalence of sleep disturbance in chronic pain." *European Review for Medical and Pharmacological Sciences* (2014); 18: 2475-2481.

4. Smith MT, et al. "Individual variation in rapid eye movement sleep is associated with pain perception in healthy women." *Sleep* (2005); 28: 809-812.

5. Zarrabian MM, et al. "Relationship between sleep, pain and disability in patients with spinal pathology." *Archives of Physical Medicine and Rehabilitation* (2014); 95: 1504-1509.

6. Agmon M and G Armon. "Increased insomnia symptoms predict the onset of back pain among employed adults." *PLOS ONE* (2014); 8: e103591. pp 1-7.

7. Baliki MN, et al. "Nociception, pain, negative moods and behavior selection." *Neuron* (2015); 87: 474-490.

8. Burns, David. *Feeling Good.* Avon Books, 1999.

9. Glasser, William. *Choice Theory: A New Psychology of Personal Freedom.* Harper Collins, 1998.

10. Trost Z, et al. "Cognitive dimensions of anger in chronic pain." *Pain* (2012); 153: 515-517.

11. Kjelsas E, et al. "Prevalence of eating disorders in female and male adolescents (14 – 15 years)." *Eating Behaviors* (2004); 5: 13-25.

12. Young AK, et al. "Assessment of presurgical psychological screening in patients undergoing spine surgery." *Journal of Spinal Disorders and Techniques*

(2014); 27: 76-79.

13.   Dement, William C, and Christopher Vaughan. *The Promise of Sleep.* Dell Publishing, 2000.

14.   Eisenberg DM, et al. "A model of integrative care for low back pain." *The Journal of Alternative and Complementary Medicine* (2012); 18: 354-362.

**Chapter 5**

1.   Frankl, Viktor. *Man's Search for Meaning.* Washington Square Press, 1959.

2.   *Committee on Advancing Pain Research, Care and Education; Institute of Medicine Relieving Pain in America: A Blueprint for Transforming Prevention, Care, Education, and Research.* The National Academies Press, 2011.

3.   Fritzell P, et al. "Lumbar fusion versus non-surgical treatment for LBP." *Spine* (2001); 26: 2521-2531.

4.   Abass A, et al. "Direct diagnosis and management of emotional factors in chronic headache patients." *Cephalgia* (2008); 28: 1305-1314.

5.   Donovan JL and DR Blake. "Patient non-compliance: deviance or reasoned decision-making?" *Social Science and Medicine* (1994); 34: 507-513.

6.   Burns, David. *Ten Days to Self-Esteem.* Harper Collins, 1993.

7.   McAbee JH, et al. "Factors associated with career satisfaction and burnout among US neurosurgeons: results of a nationwide survey." *Journal of Neurosurgery* (2015); 123: 1-13.

8.   De Mello, Anthony. *The Way to Love.* Doubleday, 1992.

9.   Blum, Deborah. *Love at Goon Park: Harry Harlow and the Science of Affection.* Perseus Publishing, 2002.

10.   Eccleston C, et al. "Patients' and professionals' understandings of the causes of chronic pain: blame, responsibility and identity protection." *Social Science & Medicine* (1997); 45: 699–709.

11.   Eisenberger N, et al. "Does social rejection hurt? An fMRI study of social exclusion." *Science* (2003); 302:290-293.

12.   Peck, Scott. *People of the Lie.* Touchstone Publishing, 1983.

**Chapter 6**

1.   Sarno, John. *Mind Over Back Pain.* Berkeley Books, 1999.

2.   Burns, David. *Feeling Good.* Avon Books, 1999.

3.   Luskin, Fred. *Forgive for Good.* HarperOne, 2003.

**Chapter 7**

1.   Evans, Patricia. *Verbal Abuse: Survivors Speak Out.* Adams Media Corporation, 1993.

2.   Wallace, Alan. Meditation retreat discussion, Spirit Rock, Woodacre, CA, 2010.

3.   DeMello, Anthony. *The Way to Love.* Doubleday, 1995.

4. Laurence, Tim. *The Hoffman Process*. Bantam, 2004.
5. Burns, David. *Feeling Good*. Avon Books, 1999.
6. Wegener, D.M., et al. "Paradoxical effects of thought suppression." *Journal of Personality and Social Psychology* (1987); 53: 5-13.
7. Deng Ming-Dao. *365 Tao: Daily Meditations*, Harper Collins, 1993.
8. Jampolsky, Gerald. *Love is Letting Go of Fear*. Random House, 2011.

**Chapter 8**

1. Azevedo C, et al. "How many neurons do you have? Some dogmas of neuroscience under revision." *European Journal of Neuroscience* (2012); 35:1-9.
2. Seminowicz DA, et al. "Effective Treatment of Chronic Low Back Pain in Humans Reverses Abnormal Brain Anatomy and Function." *The Journal of Neuroscience* (2011); 31: 7540-7550.
3. Doidge, Norman. *The Brain that Changes Itself*. Penguin Books, 2007.
4. Hashmi JA, et al. "Shape shifting pain: chronification of back pain shifts brain representation from nociceptive to emotional circuits." *Brain* (2013); 136: 2751-2768.
5. Mansour AR, et al. "Chronic pain: The role of learning and brain plasticity." *Restorative Neurology and Neuroscience* (2014); 32: 129-139.
6. Chen X, et al. "Stress enhances muscle nociceptor activity in the rat." *Neuroscience* (2011); 185: 166–173
7. Baikie K, et al. "Emotional and physical health benefits of expressive writing." *Advances in Psychiatric Treatment* (2005); 11: 338-346.
8. Wegener DM, et al. "Paradoxical effects of thought suppression." *Journal of Personality and Social Psychology* (1987); 53: 5-13.
9. Wegner DM. "The Seed of Our Undoing." *Psychological Science Agenda* (1999); Jan/Feb, 10-11.
10. Hulbert J, et al. "Inducing amnesia through systemic suppression." *Nature Communications* (2016); DOI.1038.
11. Garland E, et al. "Thought suppression as a mediator of the association between depressed mood and prescription opioid craving among chronic pain patients." Journal of Behavioral Medicine (2016); 39: 128-138.
12. Kahneman, Daniel. *Thinking Fast and Slow*. Farrar, Straus and Giroux, 2011.
13. Burns, David. *Feeling Good*. Avon Books, 1999.
14. Yancey, Philip and Paul Brand. *Pain: The Gift Nobody Wants*. DIANE Publishing Company, 1999.
15. Baliki MN and AV Apkarian. Nociception, pain, negative moods, and behavior selection. *Neuron* (2015); 87: 474-491.

**Chapter 9**

1. Bruns D and JM Disorbio. "The psychological evaluation of patients with chronic pain: a review of BHI 2 clinical and forensic interpretive consider-

ations." *Psychological Injury and Law* (2014); 7: 335–361.

2. Schug SA, et al. "Chronic pain after surgery or injury." *Pain: Clinical Updates* (2011); 19: 1-5.

3. Young AK, et al. "Assessment of presurgical psychological screening in patients undergoing spine surgery. *Journal of Spinal Disorders* (2014); 27: 76-79.

4. Luskin, Fred. *Forgive for Good.* Harper Collins, 2002.

5. Garland E, et al. "Thought suppression as a mediator of the association between depressed mood and prescription opioid craving among chronic pain patients." *Journal of Behavorial Medicine* (2016); 39: 128–138.

6. Gill KM, et al. "Social support and pain behavior." *Pain* (1987); 29: 209-217.

7. Ferrari R and AS Russell. "Effect of a symptom diary on symptom frequency and intensity in healthy subjects." *The Journal of Rheumatology* (2010); 37: 11; doi:10.3899/jrheum.100513.

## Chapter 10

1. Rahe RH, et al. "Social stress and illness onset." *Journal of Psychosomatic Research* (1964); 8: 35.

2. van Mier H, et al. "Changes in brain activity during motor learning and measured with PET: Effects of hand of performance and practice." *Journal of Neurophysiology* (1998); 80:2177-2199.

3. Burns, David. *Feeling Good,* Avon Books1999.

4. Baike KA and K Wilhelm. "Emotional and physical health benefits of expressive writing." *Advances in Psychiatric Treatment* (2005); 11:338-346.

5. Pennebaker JW & SK Beall. "Confronting a traumatic event: Toward an understanding of inhibition and disease." *Journal of Abnormal Psychology* (1986); 95: 274–281.

6. Smyth JM and J Pennebaker. "Exploring the boundary conditions of expressive writing: In search of the right recipe." *British Journal of Health Psychology* (2008); 13: 1-7.

7. Wallace, Alan. Lecture at Spirit Rock Meditation Center (2012); Woodacre, CA, 2012.

## Chapter 11

1. Centers for Disease Control and Prevention. "Trends in aging – United States and worldwide." *Morbidity and Mortality Weekly Report* (2003); 52: 101-104.

2. Trost Z, et al. "Cognitive Dimensions of anger in chronic pain." *Pain* (2012); 153: 515-517.

3. Burns, David. *Feeling Good,* Avon Books, 1999.

4. Luskin, Fred. *Forgive for Good.* Harper Collins, 2002.

5. Abass A, et al. "Direct diagnosis and management of emotional factors in chronic headache patients." *Cephalgia* (2008); 28: 1305-1314.

## Chapter 12

1. Felitti VJ, et al. "The relationship of adult health status to childhood abuse and household dysfunction." *American Journal of Preventive Medicine* (1998); 14: 245-258.
2. Gordon, Thomas. *Parent Effectiveness Training.* Three Rivers Press, 2000.
3. Hyde School, 616 High St. Bath, ME, 04530.
4. Winston, Stephanie. *The Organized Executive.* Warner Books, 2001.
5. Allen, David. *Getting Things Done.* Penguin Books, 2001.

## Chapter 13

1. Lebell, Sharon. *The Art of Living.* Harper Collins, 1995.
2. Laurence, Tim. *The Hoffman Process.* Bantam, 2004.

## Chapter 14

1. Dement, William C, and Christopher Vaughan. *The Promise of Sleep.* Dell Publishing, 2000.
2. Karaman S, et al. "Prevalence of sleep disturbance in chronic pain." *European Review for Medical and Pharmacological Sciences* (2014); 18: 2475-2481.
3. Agmon M and G Armon. "Increased insomnia symptoms predict the onset of back pain among employed adults." *PLOS ONE* (2014); 9: 1-7.
4. Hossain J, and CM Shapiro. "The prevalence, cost implications, and management of sleep disorders: An Overview." *Sleep and Breathing* (2002); 6: 85-102.
5. Zarrabian MM, et al. "Relationship between sleep, pain, and disability in patients with spinal pathology." *Archives of Physical Medicine and Rehabilitation* (2014); 95:1504-1509.
6. Van der Heijden KB, et al. "Sleep hygiene and actigraphically evaluated sleep characteristics in children with ADHD and chronic sleep onset insomnia." *Journal of Sleep Research* (2006); 15, 55-62.
7. Kryger, Meir H, Thomas Roth, and William C. Dement. *Principles and Practice of Sleep Medicine.* Saunders, 2000.
8. Harvey A and C Farrell. "The efficacy of a Pennebaker-like writing intervention for poor sleepers." *Behavioral Sleep Medicine* (2003); 2: 115-124.
9. Yang P, et al. "Exercise training improves sleep quality in middle-aged and older adults with sleep problems: a systematic review." *Journal of Physiotherapy* (2012); 58: 157-163.
10. Gould RL, et al. "Interventions for reducing benzodiazepine use in older people: Meta-analysis of randomized controlled trials." *The British Journal of Psychiatry* (2014); 204: 98-107.
11. Manber R, et al. "Cognitive behavioral therapy for insomnia enhances depression outcome in patients with comorbid major depressive disorder and insomnia." *Sleep* (2008); 3: 489-495.
12. Burns, David. *Feeling Good.* Avon Books, 1999.

13. Bruflat AK, et al. "Stress management as an adjunct to physical therapy for chronic neck pain." *Physical Therapy* (2012); 92:1348-1359.

14. Hunt MA, et al. "A physiotherapist-delivered, combined exercise and pain coping skills training intervention for individuals with knee osteoarthritis: a pilot study." *Knee* (2013); 20:106-112.

15. Felitti VJ, et al. "The relationship of adult health status to childhood abuse and family dysfunction." *American Journal of Preventive Medicine* (1998), 14: 245-258.

16. Chapman, D, et al. "Adverse childhood experiences and sleep disturbances in adults." *Sleep Medicine* (2011); 12: 773-779.

17. Hulbert JC, et al. "Inducing amnesia through systemic suppression." *Nature Communications* (2016); 11:1-9.

**Chapter 15**

1. Liang D, et al. "Chronic morphine administration enhances nociceptive sensitivity and local cytokine production after incision." *Molecular Pain* (2008); 4:7.

2. Drendel A, et al. "A randomized clinical trial of ibuprofen versus acetamino-phen and codeine in pediatric arm fractures." *Annals of Emergency Medicine* (2009); Oct: 533-60.

**Chapter 16**

1. Giesecke T, et al. "Evidence of augmented central pain processing in idio-pathic chronic low back pain." *Arthritis and Rheumatism* (2004); 50: 613-623.

2. Safren SA, et al. "Cognitive behavioral therapy for adherence and depression (CBTAD) in HIV-infected injection drug users: a randomized controlled trial." Journal of Consulting and Clinical Psychology (2012); 80: 404-415

3. Louis Harris and Associates. *The Perrier Study: Fitness in America*. Great Waters of France, 1979.

4. Felitti VJ, et al. "The relationship of adult health status to childhood abuse and family dysfunction." *American Journal of Preventive Medicine* (1998), 14: 245-258.

5. Lucas, DB, and B Bresler. "Stability of the Ligamentous Spine." *Biomechanics Laboratory Report 40*, San Francisco: University of California, 1961.

6. Centers for Disease Control and Prevention. "Trends in aging – United States and worldwide." *Morbidity and Mortality Weekly Report* (2003); 52: 101-104.

7. Edwards RR, et al. "Pain, catastrophizing, and depression in the rheumatic diseases." *Nature Reviews Rheumatology* (2011); 7: 216-224.

**Chapter 17**

1. Dalai Lama and Howard Cutler. *The Art of Happiness, 10th Anniversary Edi-tion: A Handbook for Living*. Riverhead Books, 1998.

2.  Frankl, Viktor. *Man's Search for Meaning.* Beacon Press, 2006.
3.  Greenblatt, Stephen. *The Swerve: How the World Became Modern.* W. W. Norton Co. 2011.
4.  Laurence, Tim. *The Hoffman Process* Bantam, 2004.
5.  Cozolino, Louis. *The Neuroscience of Human Relationships.* W. W. Norton & Company, 2014.

## Appendix A

1.  Carragee EJ, et al. "A gold standard evaluation of the 'discogenic pain' diagnosis as determined by provocative discography." *Spine* (2006) 31:2115-2123.
2.  Franklin GM, et al. "Outcomes of lumbar fusion in Washington state workers' compensation." *Spine* (2994); 19: 1897–1903; discussion 1904
3.  Buchbinder R, et al. "Doctors with a special interest in back pain have poorer knowledge about how to treat back pain." *Spine* (2009); 34: 1218-1226.
4.  Young AK, et al. "Assessment of presurgical psychological screening in patients undergoing spine surgery." *Journal of Spinal Disorders & Techniques* (2014); 27: 76-79.
5.  Harris G. "Talk doesn't pay, so psychiatry turns instead to drug therapy." New York Times, March 6, 2011.
6.  Nguyen TH, et al. "Long-term outcomes of lumbar fusion among Workers' Compensation subjects." *Spine* (2011); 36:320-331.
7.  Martin BI, et al. "Reoperation rates following lumbar spine surgery and the influence of spinal fusion procedures." *Spine* (2007); 32: 382-387.
8.  Fritzell P, et al. "Lumbar fusion versus non-surgical treatment for chronic low back pain: a multicenter randomized controlled trial from the Swedish Lumbar Spine Study Group." *Spine* (2001); 26: 2521-2532.
9.  Perkins FM and H Kehlet. "Chronic Pain as an Outcome of Surgery." *Anesthesiology* (2000); 93: 1123-1133.

# Recommended Reading

## STRONGLY RECOMMENDED

- *The Talent Code: Greatness Isn't Born. It's Grown. Here's How.* by Daniel Coyle
- *Feeling Good: The New Mood Therapy* by David Burns, MD
- *Forgive for Good: A Proven Prescription for Health and Happiness* by Fred Luskin, PhD
- *Getting Things Done: The Art of Stress-Free Productivity* by David Allen
- *Unlearn Your Pain* by Howard Schubiner, MD, with Michael Betzold
- *Parent Effectiveness Training: The Proven Program for Raising Responsible Children* by Thomas Gordon, MD
- *The Art of Living: The Classical Manual on Virtue, Happiness, and Effectiveness* by Epictetus (modern translation by Sharon Lebell)
- *The Way to Love: The Last Meditations of Anthony de Mello* by Anthony de Mello
- *Verbal Abuse: Survivors Speak Out* by Patricia Evans
- *Journey into Love: Ten Steps to Wholeness* by Kani Comstock & Marisa Thame
- *8 Steps to a Pain-Free Back: Natural Posture Solutions for Pain in the Back, Neck, Shoulder, Hip, Knee, and Foot (Remember When It Didn't Hurt)* by Esther Gokhale

## Books of Interest

- *Man's Search for Meaning* by Viktor Frankl, MD, PhD
- *Pain: The Gift that Nobody Wants* by Paul Brand, MD
- *The Swerve: How the World Became Modern* by Stephen Greenblatt, PhD

## Websites

- www.backincontrol.com

# Helpful Organizations

### Hyde Schools

Hyde Schools is a network of public and boarding schools and programs known widely for its successful and unique approach to helping students develop character. Parental involvement is a key factor in Hyde's reputation as one of the premiere character-building schools in the world. I acquired many of the concepts in this book while attending Hyde with my daughter. Hyde represents the next step in the evolution of education in this country.

### Hoffman Institute

The Hoffman Quadrinity Process is based on the principle that the persistent negative behaviors, moods, and attitudes we experience as adults have their roots in our childhood. Until pain from childhood is resolved, it dominates our adult lives (thoughts, emotions, and actions), whether or not we are aware of it. The Hoffman Process is designed to heal and transform negative, self-defeating patterns and bring about a powerful realignment and integration of the four fundamental dimensions of our being: intellect, emotions, body, and spirit. The Hoffman Quadrinity Process uses a combination of proven techniques that include guided visualization, journaling, and cathartic work. I attended the Hoffman Institute in 2009, and its teachings significantly influenced the writing of this book, giving me the tools to finish it.

### Strozzi Institute

I have learned that you cannot calm your mind with your mind but you can calm your mind with your body. Richard Strozzi-Heckler is a remarkable psychologist who employs a mind-body approach to teach leadership. The Strozzi Institute is located in Petaluma, CA, and offers coaching services in leadership training, organizational development, and personal mastery. Dr. Strozzi-Heckler is well-versed in the martial art of aikido, whose principles he brings to his teaching. His tools are useful in both calming your mind and creating your vision to live life without pain.